From the Ground VEGAN COOKBOOK

Mechille Renee Tate-Akinkuotu

Bledsoe Publishing Company LLC

Library of Congress Cataloging-in-Publication Data has been applied for.

ISBN: 978-1-957551-31-9 (Paperback); 978-1-957551-32-6 (eBook)
Cover Design by: Innovara Design Studio LLC
Interior Design by: Innovara Design Studio LLC
Published by: Bledsoe Publishing Company LLC
Printed in the United States of America

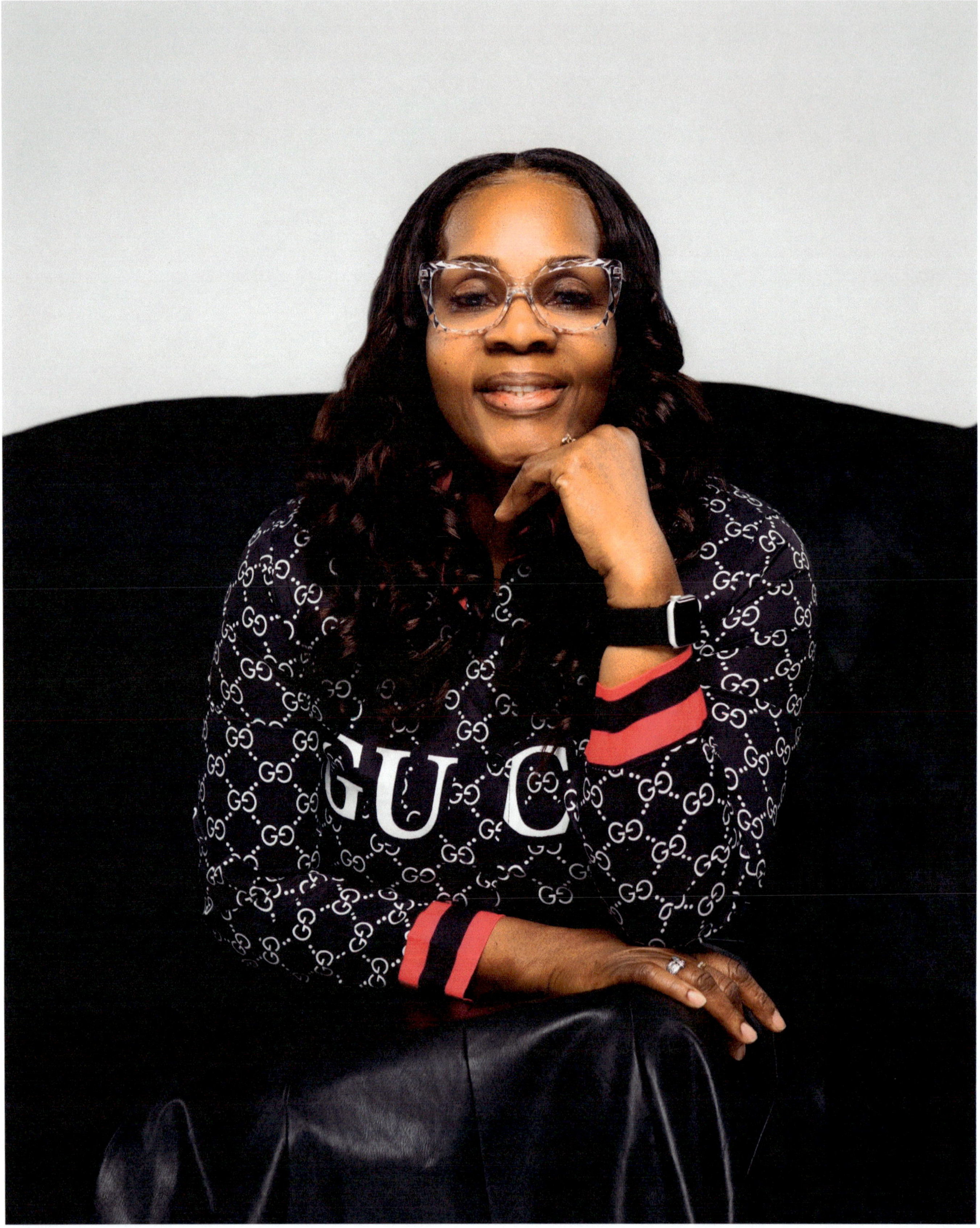

MESSAGE FROM THE AUTHOR

Hello, my name is Mechille Renee Tate-Akinkuotu, and my decision to become vegan was deeply rooted in faith, prayer, and a commitment to my health. I knew I did not want to spend the rest of my life dependent on pills or insulin to manage diabetes. High blood pressure and high cholesterol were real threats, and the way I was eating was leading me down a dangerous path. I was slowly harming my own body with every meal, and I knew it was time to make a change.

I committed to a 40-day fast, consuming only fruits, vegetables, and water while staying grounded in prayer. I eliminated meat, refined sugars, and processed foods, choosing instead to nourish my body with natural, wholesome ingredients. At the start of my journey, my A1C was a staggering 12%, my blood pressure was 158/101, and I was taking six different medications every morning.

Now, ten months later, I have reclaimed my health. My A1C is now 4%, meaning I am no longer diabetic. My blood pressure is a healthy 123/78, and my cholesterol levels are within normal range. But beyond the medical numbers, I feel better than ever. I have energy, I can run without struggling, and I sleep soundly through the night.

This journey has reshaped the way I view food. I now see it as nourishment and fuel rather than comfort or convenience. Every meal I prepare is intentional, focused on feeding my body what it needs to thrive. If you are looking for a way to step into a healthier way of living, my cookbook is for you. It is filled with flavorful, satisfying meals that will support your health while allowing you to truly enjoy what you eat.

Your health is in your hands, and every meal is an opportunity to choose better. I invite you to join me on this journey. May this book bless you, and may your wellness flourish!

— Mechille Renee Tate-Akinkuotu

INTRODUCTION

Food is more than just something we eat; it is a reflection of who we are, where we come from, and how we care for ourselves. Adopting a plant-based lifestyle has been an eye-opening journey. One that has deepened my connection to health, wellness, and the power of mindful eating. There was a time when convenience and habits dictated my food choices, but as I learned more about nutrition and the impact of food on the body, I realized that the way I nourish myself affects every part of my life. Food has the power to energize, to heal, and to sustain, but only if we choose it with intention.

Making the shift to plant-based eating is not about restriction; it is about abundance. It is about discovering the richness of nature's offerings, the vibrant flavors of fresh produce, and the satisfying nourishment that comes from whole, unprocessed foods. It is a journey of reconnecting with real food, moving away from what has been mass-produced and marketed as "healthy," and returning to what truly fuels our bodies. The more I explored this way of eating, the more I realized how much misinformation exists about plant-based living. Some believe it is too expensive, too complicated, or too bland, but that could not be further from the truth. With the right knowledge and preparation, plant-based meals are not only accessible but deeply flavorful and fulfilling. The key is learning how to build balanced, delicious meals that satisfy both the body and the soul. Whether it is a hearty lentil soup, a protein-packed grain bowl, or a flavorful vegetable stir-fry, the possibilities are endless.

But this journey is not just about food, it is about self-care, discipline, and making choices that align with long-term well-being. It is about understanding that food is medicine and that what we eat directly impacts our energy, mood, and overall quality of life. It is about learning to listen to the body's needs and honoring the body with ingredients that nourish rather than deplete. Making mindful choices in the kitchen extends into all aspects of life, fostering a sense of clarity, purpose, and empowerment.

The goal of the *From the Ground Vegan Cookbook* is to share the vegan lifestyle in a way that is inviting, practical, and enjoyable. This is not a diet; it is a shift in perspective, an opportunity to embrace a way of eating that enhances life in ways that go far beyond the plate. By educating ourselves and making small, intentional changes, we can redefine what it means to eat well. Through this journey, I hope this cookbook inspires others to see food not just as something to consume but as a tool for creating healthy habits, healing, and joy.

TABLE OF CONTENTS

VEGAN Drinks

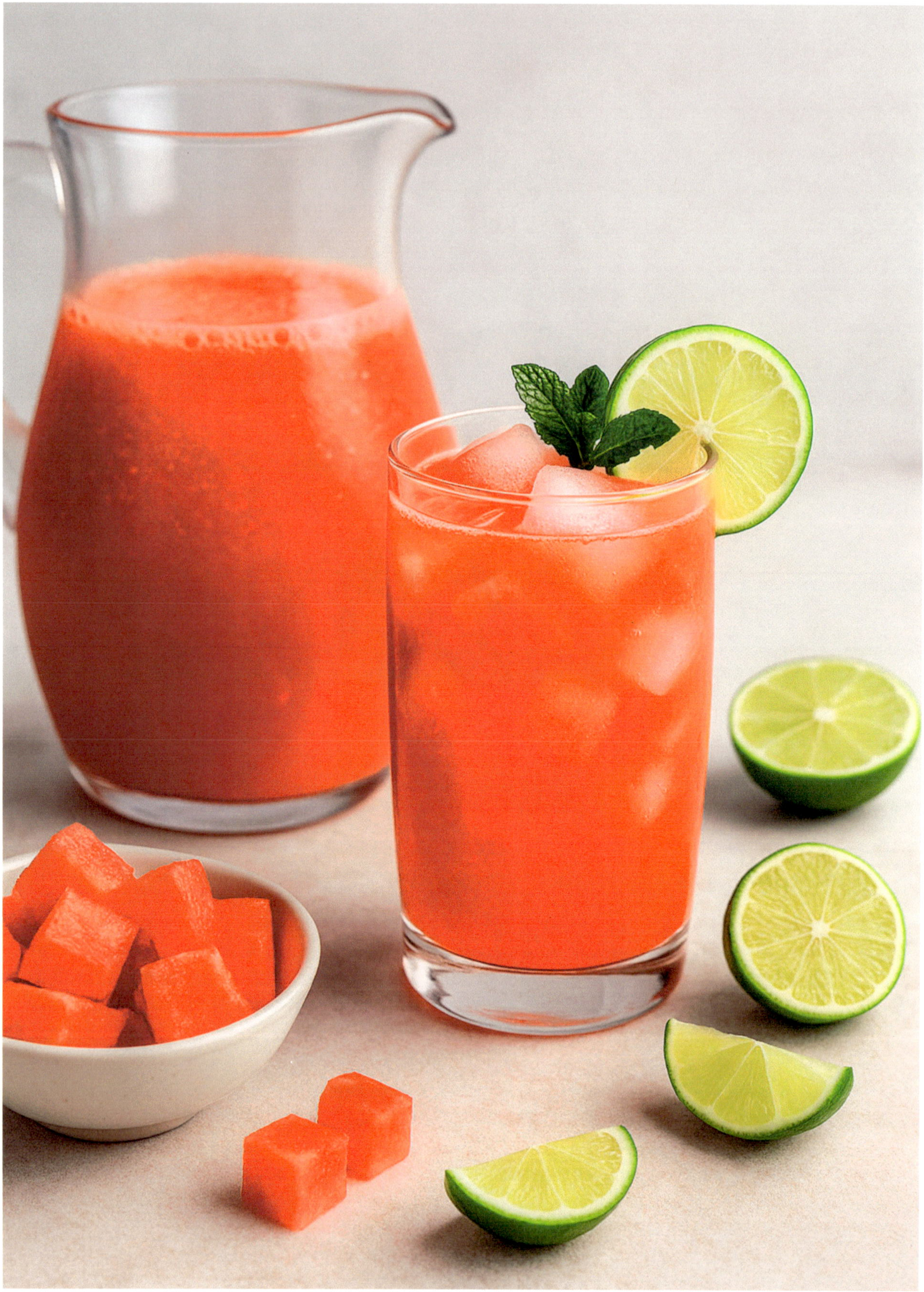

VEGAN WATERMELON JUICE

This refreshing vegan watermelon juice is simple, hydrating, and packed with flavor. The sweetness of watermelon is perfectly balanced by the tanginess of lime and the slight kick from fresh ginger. This juice is ideal for rehydration, detoxification, weight loss and healing.

INGREDIENTS

- 4 cups watermelon (cubed, seedless)
- 1-2 limes (juiced)
- 1-inch piece of fresh ginger (peeled and grated or finely chopped)
- Ice (optional)

INSTRUCTIONS

Prepare the Ingredients

1. **Cut the Watermelon**: Cut a seedless watermelon into cubes and measure about 4 cups.
2. **Juice the Limes**: Squeeze the juice from 1-2 limes (depending on how tangy you like it) and set aside.
3. **Grate the Ginger**: Peel and grate a 1-inch piece of fresh ginger.

Blend the Juice

1. **Add Ingredients to Blender**: Place the cubed watermelon, lime juice, and grated ginger into a blender.
2. **Blend**: Blend on high until everything is well combined and smooth.
   - If you prefer a smoother texture, you can strain the juice through a fine mesh sieve or cheesecloth to remove any pulp, but this step is optional.

Serve

1. **Chill and Serve**: Pour the watermelon juice into a glass filled with ice if you like it cold. Stir well and enjoy!
   - **Optional Garnish**: You can garnish the juice with a lime wedge or mint leaves for added freshness.

HEALING AND NUTRITION

This vegan watermelon juice is not only incredibly hydrating and refreshing but also a powerful aid in healing and weight loss. Watermelon is made up of about 90% water, making it one of the best fruits for hydration and detoxification. It's also low in calories, yet rich in essential nutrients like vitamins A, C, and antioxidants that help reduce inflammation and support overall health.

One person shared how they incorporated this watermelon juice into their daily routine as a way to stay hydrated and control cravings during their weight loss journey. By sipping on this juice throughout the day, they felt more energized and less prone to snacking between meals. The ginger in the juice also helped boost their digestion and metabolism, further supporting their weight loss goals.

Over the course of two months, they lost 6 pounds, partly thanks to this juice, which became their go-to drink for staying refreshed and healthy. They also noticed improvements in their skin, as the antioxidants in watermelon helped reduce bloating and flush out toxins. Lime, being rich in vitamin C, boosted their immune system, while ginger added anti-inflammatory benefits, soothing their digestive system and enhancing fat-burning processes.

This simple yet nutrient-packed watermelon juice is a perfect addition to any diet for those looking to promote healing and support healthy weight loss naturally!

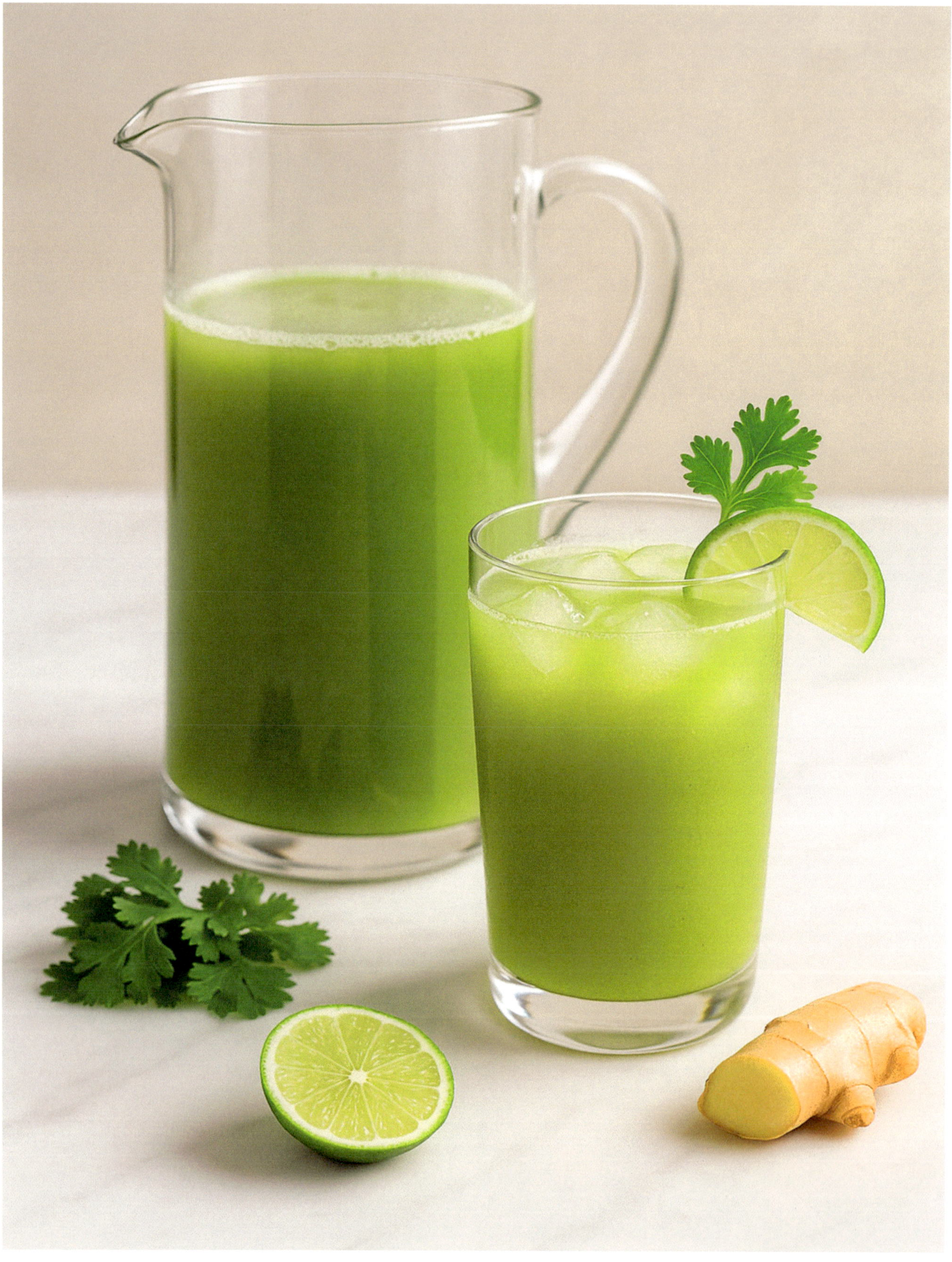

VEGAN JUST JUICY JUICE

INGREDIENTS:

- 1-inch piece of fresh ginger (peeled)
- Juice of 2 limes
- 1 cup fresh orange juice (about 2-3 oranges)
- A handful of fresh cilantro leaves
- 1/4 cup water (optional for thinning)
- Ice cubes (optional)

INSTRUCTIONS:

Prepare the Ingredients

1. **Peel and grate** the fresh ginger or cut it into small pieces for easier blending.
2. **Juice the limes** and oranges. You can use a hand juicer or electric juicer for fresh citrus juice. Set the juice aside.
3. **Rinse the cilantro** thoroughly and pick off the leaves, discarding the stems.

Blend the Juice

1. In a blender, combine the grated ginger, lime juice, orange juice, and cilantro leaves.
2. **Blend** on high for about 30-60 seconds, or until all ingredients are well combined and the cilantro is finely chopped.
3. If you prefer a thinner consistency, add up to 1/4 cup of water and blend again.

Strain (Optional)

1. If you prefer a smooth juice, you can strain the mixture through a fine mesh sieve to remove the pulp.

Serve

1. Pour the juice over ice cubes if desired or chill in the refrigerator before serving.
2. Garnish with a sprig of cilantro or a slice of lime and enjoy this refreshing and zesty vegan juice!

HEALING AND NUTRITION

This **Just Juicy Juice** recipe is a powerhouse of nutrients that aids digestion, boosts the immune system, and supports weight loss. **Ginger** is known for its anti-inflammatory and digestive benefits, helping to reduce bloating, improve gut health, and increase metabolism. Its warming properties also promote detoxification and fat burning, making it a great addition to weight-loss diets.

Lime and **orange juice** are rich in vitamin C, which boosts immunity, fights free radicals, and promotes collagen production. The citrusy elements of the juice also act as natural diuretics, helping to flush out toxins and excess water weight from the body.

Cilantro, often underestimated, is a powerful detoxifier. It helps to remove heavy metals from the body, aids digestion, and contains antioxidants that support overall health. For those looking to shed excess pounds, cilantro helps boost metabolism and improve digestion, preventing sluggishness.

By incorporating this fresh, nutrient-dense juice into their routine, many people have experienced reduced bloating, increased energy levels, and enhanced fat burning. It's a natural, refreshing way to support the body's detoxification processes while staying hydrated and nourished. This juice makes an excellent addition to any weight-loss regimen or healing journey, providing both cleansing and replenishing benefits.

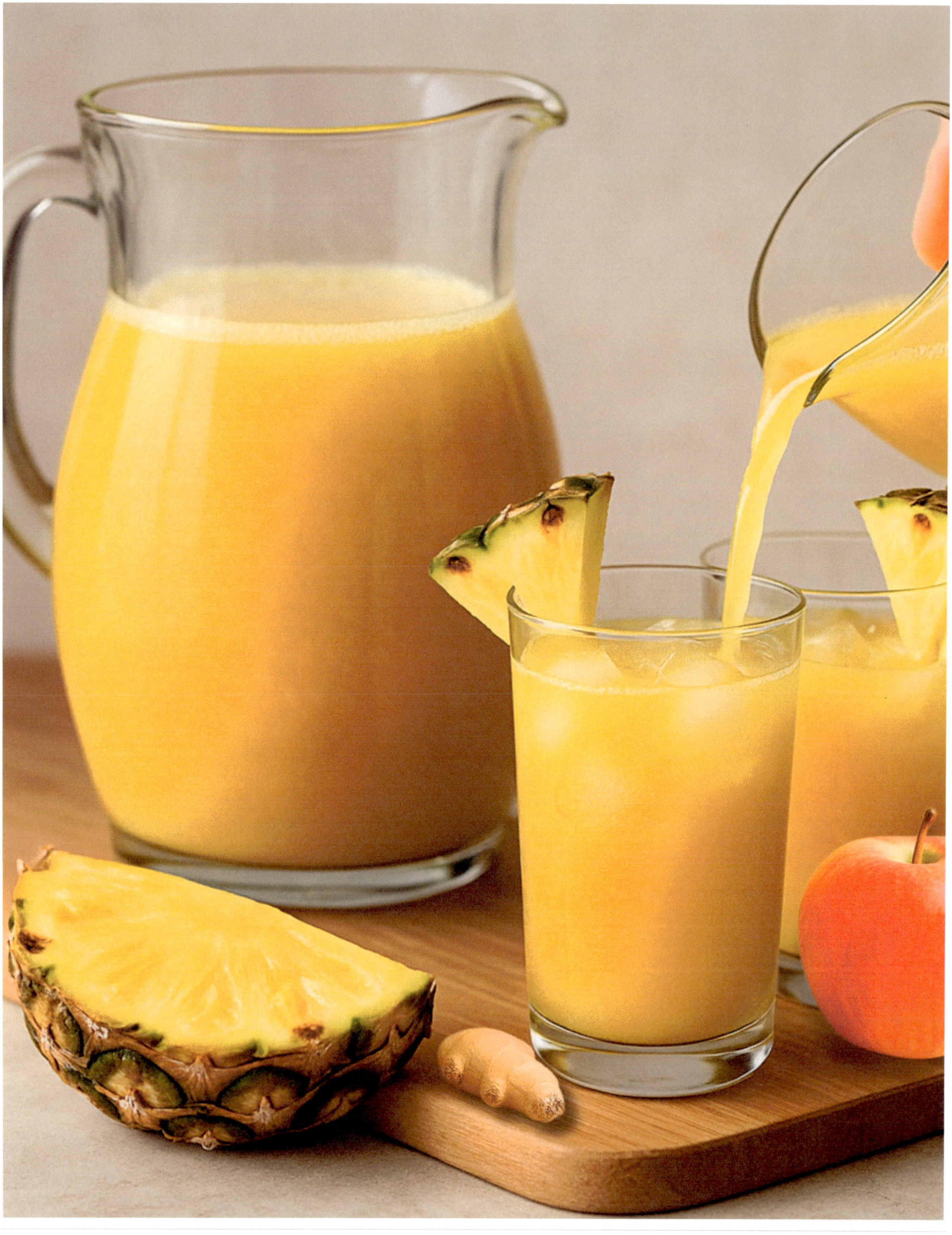

VEGAN PINEAPPLE APPLE GINGER JUICE

INGREDIENTS:

- 1/2 medium pineapple (peeled and chopped)
- 2 medium apples (cored and chopped, use a sweet variety like Fuji or Gala)
- 1-inch piece of fresh ginger (peeled)
- 1/4 cup water (optional for thinning)
- Ice cubes (optional)

INSTRUCTIONS:

Prepare the Ingredients

1. **Peel and chop** the pineapple into chunks.
2. **Core and chop** the apples into pieces, leaving the skin on for extra fiber.
3. **Peel and slice** the ginger into smaller pieces for easier blending or juicing.

Blend or Juice

Blender Method:

1. Place the pineapple, apple, ginger, and water (if using) into a high-speed blender.
2. Blend on high until all the ingredients are fully combined and smooth, about 1-2 minutes.
3. If you prefer a smooth juice, strain the mixture using a fine mesh sieve or nut milk bag to remove the pulp.

Juicer Method:

1. If you have a juicer, feed the pineapple, apple, and ginger through the juicer.
2. Collect the fresh juice and stir well.

Serve

1. Pour the juice into glasses over ice cubes for a chilled, refreshing drink.
2. Garnish with a slice of pineapple or apple for presentation, and enjoy your tropical, tangy juice!

HEALING AND NUTRITION

This Pineapple Apple Ginger juice is packed with powerful ingredients that not only taste amazing but also offer significant health benefits. **Pineapple** contains bromelain, an enzyme known for its anti-inflammatory and digestive benefits. It helps break down proteins, improving digestion and reducing bloating. Both of which are essential for weight loss. Pineapple is also low in calories and rich in vitamin C, boosting immunity and helping the body metabolize fat.

Apples are high in fiber and water content, which aids in weight management by promoting satiety and reducing overall calorie intake. Apples also help in regulating blood sugar, which is essential for preventing insulin spikes that can lead to weight gain. The skin of apples provides extra fiber, supporting digestive health and keeping you full longer.

Ginger is a metabolism-boosting superfood. Known for its thermogenic effects, it helps the body burn more calories by stimulating fat burning. Ginger also promotes gut health, relieves indigestion, and reduces inflammation, making it an excellent addition to any weight-loss or detox regimen.

People who have incorporated this juice into their daily routine have reported reduced bloating, improved digestion, and increased energy levels. It is a refreshing taste with nutritional benefits that makes it a perfect companion for weight loss and overall healing. With the combination of **pineapple's cleansing enzymes**, **apple's fiber-rich goodness**, and **ginger's fat-burning properties**, this juice can serve as a delicious and healthy way to support a balanced diet and boost metabolism naturally.

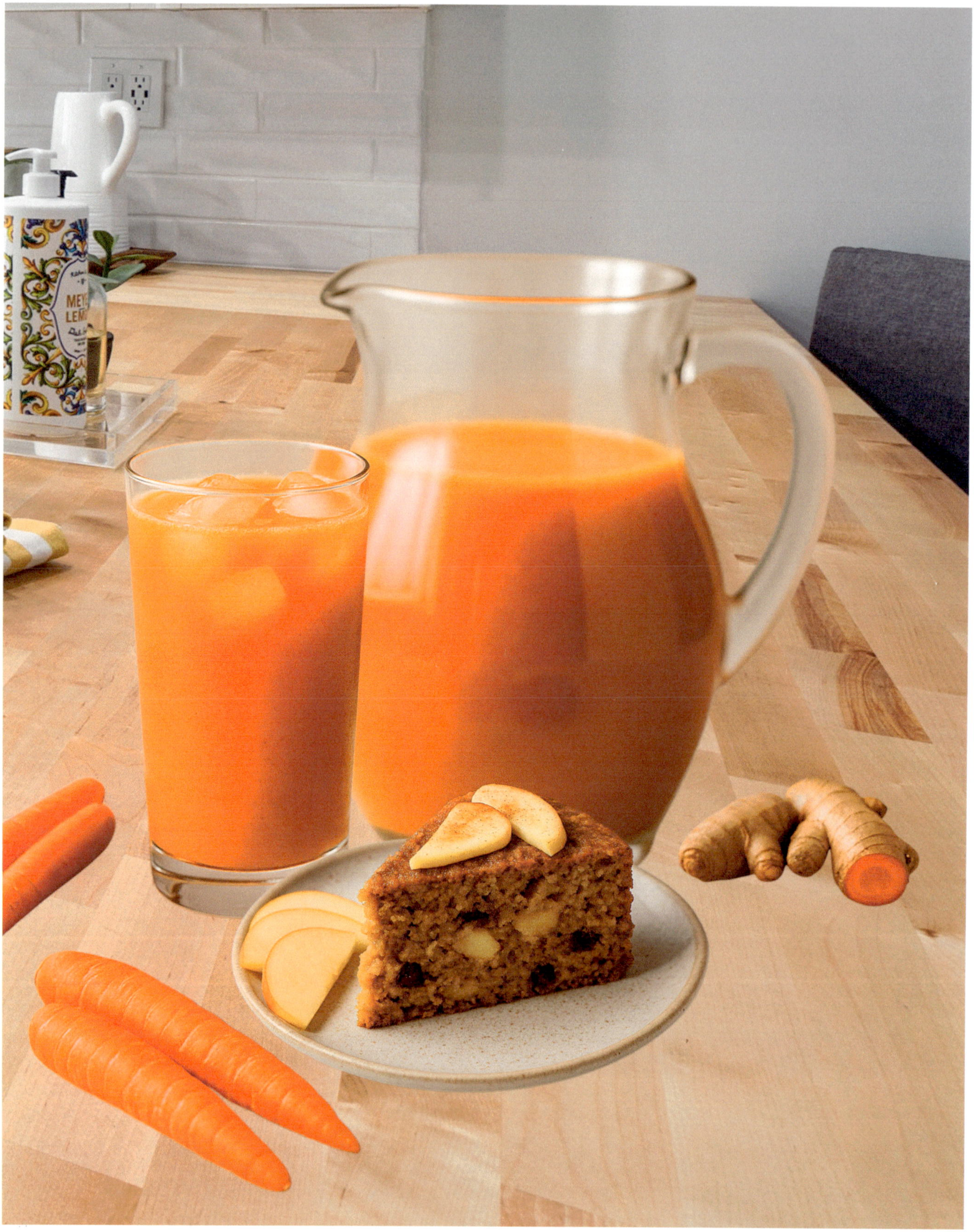

VEGAN CARROT GINGER TURMERIC JUICE

INGREDIENTS:

- 4 large carrots (peeled and chopped)
- 1-inch piece of fresh ginger (peeled)
- 1-inch piece of fresh turmeric root (peeled) or 1 teaspoon ground turmeric
- A pinch of black pepper (to activate the curcumin in turmeric)
- 1/4 cup water (optional, for thinning the juice)
- Ice cubes (optional)

INSTRUCTIONS:

Prepare the Ingredients

1. **Peel and chop the carrots** into smaller pieces for easier blending or juicing.
2. **Peel the ginger and turmeric root**, cutting them into smaller slices to help them blend well.
3. **Measure out a pinch of black pepper**, which will help the body absorb turmeric's beneficial compounds.

Blend or Juice

Blender Method:

1. Place the chopped carrots, ginger, turmeric, black pepper, and water into a high-speed blender.
2. Blend on high until smooth, for about 1-2 minutes.
3. If you prefer a smooth juice, strain the mixture using a fine mesh sieve or a nut milk bag to remove the pulp.

Juicer Method:

1. If you have a juicer, feed the carrots, ginger, and turmeric through the juicer.
2. Add a pinch of black pepper to the finished juice and stir well.

Serve

1. Pour the juice into a glass over ice cubes, if desired, for a chilled drink.
2. Stir well and enjoy your vibrant, earthy, and anti-inflammatory juice!

HEALING AND NUTRITION

This **Carrot Ginger Turmeric Juice** is a nutrient-packed powerhouse that supports both healing and weight loss. **Carrots** are rich in beta-carotene, which converts to vitamin A in the body, supporting eye health, skin repair, and immune function. Their natural sweetness also makes this juice delicious while remaining low in calories, promoting healthy digestion and satiety without excess sugar intake.

Ginger adds a spicy kick while promoting digestion, relieving bloating, and stimulating metabolism. It has thermogenic properties that can help the body burn more calories, making it an excellent ingredient for weight loss efforts. Ginger also fights inflammation, reducing symptoms like water retention and swelling.

Turmeric is one of the most potent anti-inflammatory foods available. Its active compound, curcumin, has been shown to improve metabolism and support fat loss. When combined with a pinch of black pepper, the absorption of curcumin increases significantly, enhancing its effectiveness in reducing inflammation and promoting overall healing in the body.

This juice is often praised by those seeking to lose weight and enhance their overall health because it not only detoxifies the body but also boosts metabolism and reduces inflammation. Many people who incorporate this juice into their diet have reported feeling lighter, more energized, and less bloated. The combination of turmeric's powerful healing properties and ginger's ability to ignite the digestive fire makes this juice a great companion on the journey to better health and weight management.

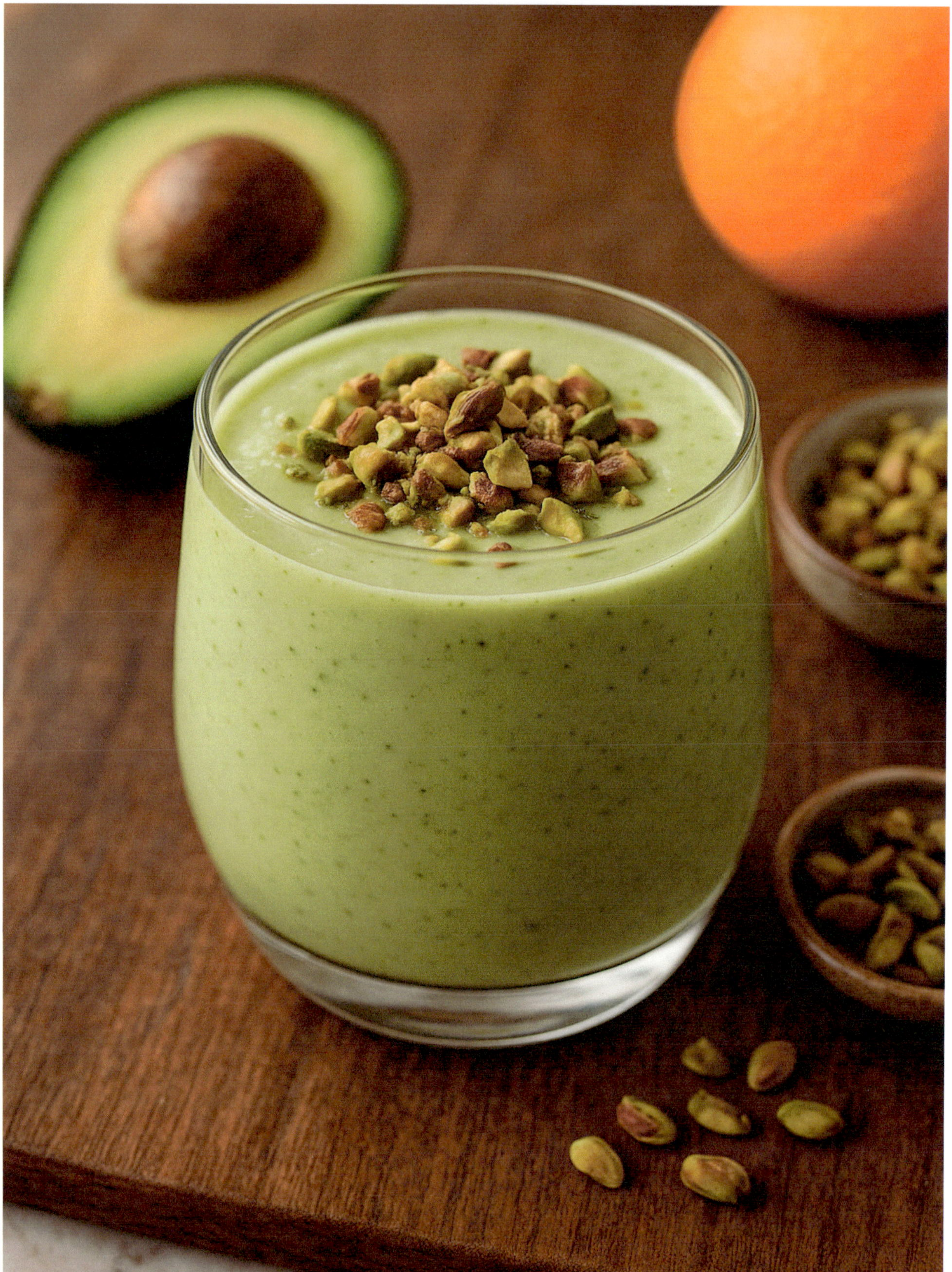

VEGAN AVOCADO SMOOTHIE

This creamy and refreshing vegan avocado smoothie combines the richness of avocado with the tangy sweetness of orange juice and the nutty crunch of pistachios. It is a perfect blend of healthy fats, vitamins, and natural sweetness, making it ideal for a nourishing snack or a light meal.

INGREDIENTS

- 1 ripe avocado
- 1 cup fresh orange juice (or more, depending on desired consistency)
- 1 tbsp organic agave syrup (or maple syrup for a fully vegan option, instead of honey)
- 2 tbsp chopped pistachios
- 4-5 ice cubes

INSTRUCTIONS

Prepare the Ingredients

- **Scoop the Avocado**: Cut the ripe avocado in half, remove the pit, and scoop out the flesh.
- **Juice the Orange**: Freshly squeeze oranges to get 1 cup of juice or use store-bought if you are in a hurry.
- **Chop the Pistachios**: Roughly chop the pistachios for adding texture to your smoothie.

Blend the Smoothie

- **Add Ingredients to Blender**: Place the avocado, orange juice, agave syrup (or maple syrup), and ice cubes into the blender.
- **Blend:** Blend on high until smooth and creamy. If you prefer a thinner consistency, you can add more orange juice.

Garnish and Serve

- **Add Pistachios**: Once the smoothie is blended, pour it into a glass and top with the chopped pistachios for a crunchy contrast.
- **Serve Immediately**: Enjoy your smoothie fresh and cold!

HEALING AND NUTRITION

This vegan avocado smoothie is not only delicious but also packed with ingredients that can support healing and weight loss. Avocados are full of heart-healthy monounsaturated fats, which help you feel full and satisfied while providing essential nutrients like potassium and fiber. These fats are known to promote fat burning and reduce belly fat while nourishing the body.

One person who regularly drank this avocado smoothie as part of their weight loss routine reported feeling more energized and fuller for longer after each serving. By swapping out high-calorie snacks with this nutrient-dense smoothie, they were able to control their appetite and reduce unnecessary snacking. Over three months, they lost 8 pounds while incorporating the avocado smoothie into their breakfast routine.

The natural sweetness from orange juice provides vitamin C, which supports immune function, while pistachios offer a satisfying crunch and additional protein, helping to curb hunger. By opting for agave syrup or maple syrup instead of refined sugars, you can enjoy a sweet yet healthier option, leading to more balanced blood sugar levels.

This smoothie is perfect for anyone looking to boost their energy, promote fat loss, and fuel their body with clean, wholesome ingredients.

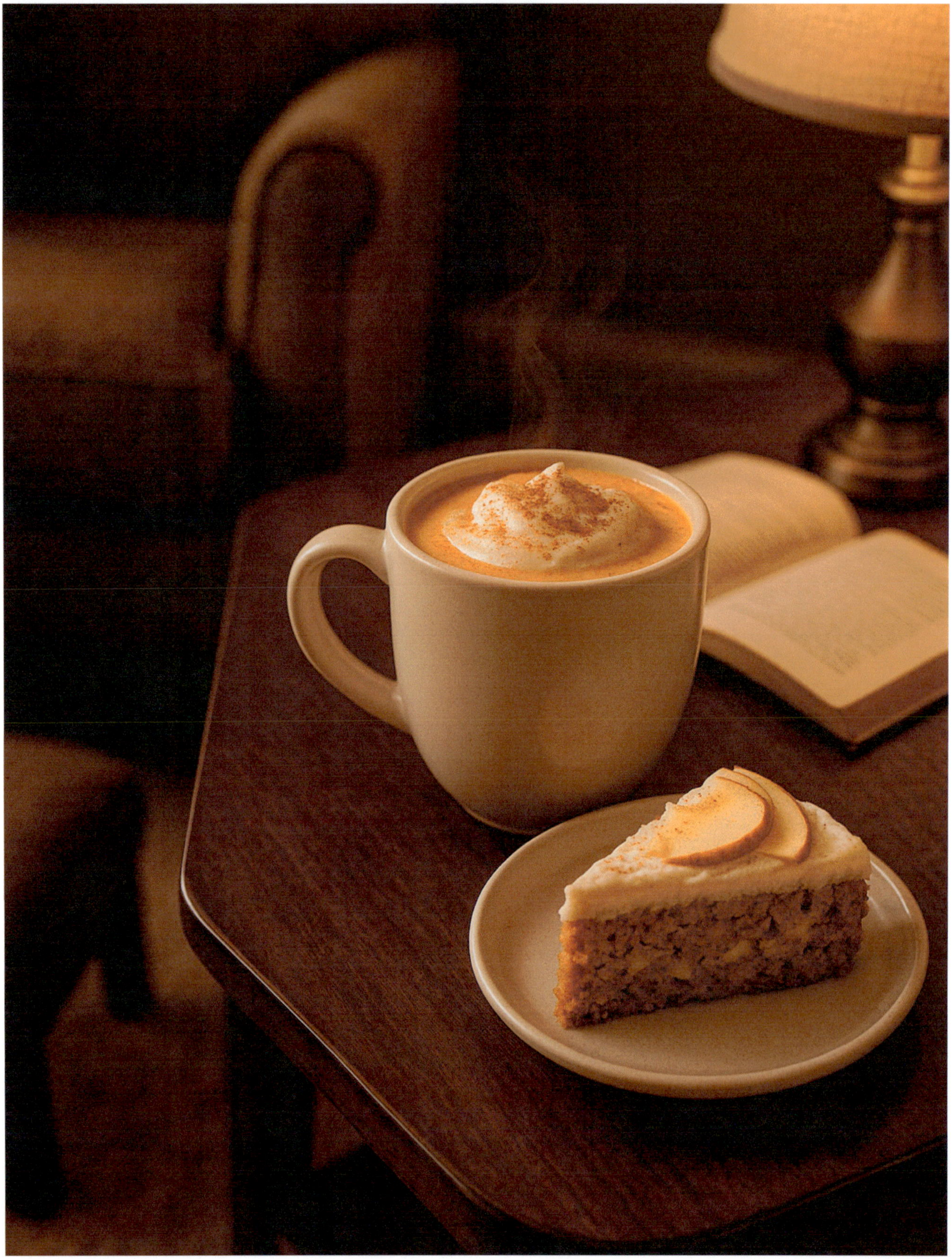

VEGAN PUMPKIN SPICE LATTE

INGREDIENTS:

For the Latte:

- 1/2 cup brewed coffee (hot or cold)
- 1/2 cup coconut milk (canned or carton)
- 1/4 cup water
- 1/4 cup organic pumpkin puree (canned or homemade)
- 1-2 tablespoons agave syrup or maple syrup (adjust to taste)
- 1/2 teaspoon vanilla extract
- 1/2 teaspoon pumpkin spice (or to taste)
- Optional: a pinch of salt (to enhance flavor)

For the Cashew Cream Topping:

- 1/2 cup raw or salted cashews (soaked in water for 2-4 hours)
- 1/2 teaspoon vanilla extract
- Water (as needed for blending)

INSTRUCTIONS:

Prepare the Cashew Cream:

- Drain and rinse the soaked cashews.
- In a high-speed blender, combine the soaked cashews, 1/2 teaspoon of vanilla extract, and a little water (about 1-2 tablespoons to start).
- Blend until smooth and creamy, adding more water as needed to achieve a whipped cream consistency, and set aside.

Make the Pumpkin Spice Latte:

- In a small saucepan, combine the coconut milk, water, organic pumpkin puree, agave or maple syrup, pumpkin spice, and a pinch of salt (if using).
- Heat the mixture over medium heat, whisking continuously until it is heated through and well combined (about 3-5 minutes). Be careful not to boil it.
- Remove from heat and add the brewed coffee. Stir well to combine.

Serve:

- Pour the pumpkin spice latte into a large mug.
- Top with a generous dollop of cashew cream.
- Sprinkle a little extra pumpkin spice on top for garnish, if desired.

Enjoy:

- Enjoy your warm, cozy pumpkin spice latte!

HEALING AND NUTRITION

This vegan pumpkin spice latte is not only delicious but also offers several health benefits that support healing and weight loss.

1. **Pumpkin** is a nutrient-dense food high in fiber, vitamins A and C, and antioxidants. Its fiber content aids digestion and helps you feel fuller for longer, which is beneficial for weight management. Additionally, the antioxidants in pumpkin can help reduce inflammation and support overall health.
2. **Cashews** provide healthy fats, protein, and essential minerals like magnesium and zinc. The healthy fats in cashews can promote heart health and help maintain a balanced diet. The creamy texture of the cashew cream also adds a satisfying richness without the unhealthy saturated fats found in dairy.
3. **Coconut milk** is rich in medium-chain triglycerides (MCTs), which may support metabolism and promote weight loss. It also adds a creamy texture and delicious flavor to the latte.
4. **Pumpkin spice** often contains cinnamon, nutmeg, and ginger, which are known for their anti-inflammatory properties and can help regulate blood sugar levels. This makes the latte not only flavorful but also beneficial for maintaining energy levels and reducing cravings.
5. **Agave or maple syrup** provides natural sweetness without the refined sugars found in many coffee shop drinks. They can satisfy your sweet tooth while offering some trace nutrients.

By choosing this vegan pumpkin spice latte, you can indulge in a seasonal favorite while nourishing your body with wholesome ingredients. It is a great way to enjoy the flavors of fall without compromising your health goals.

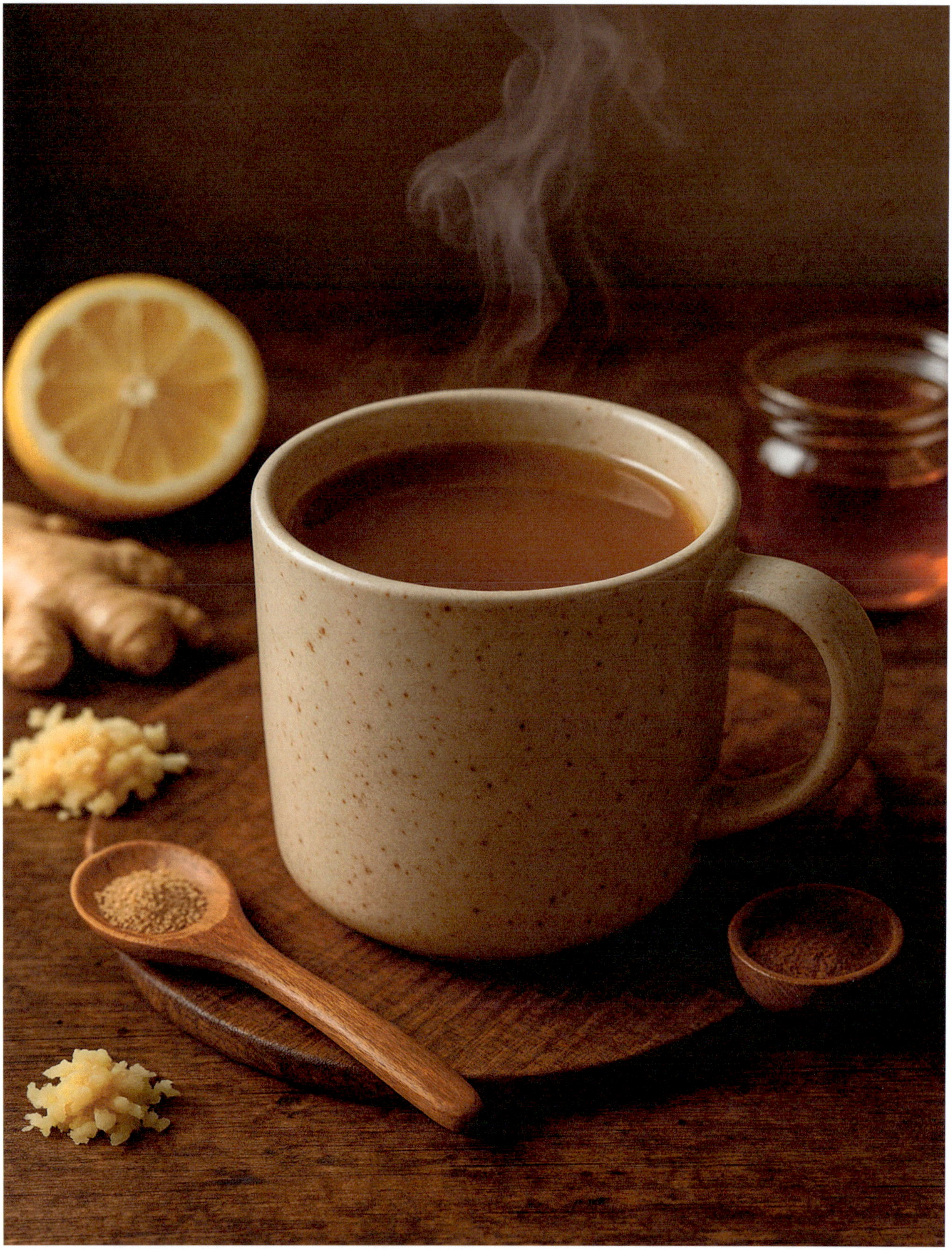

VEGAN HERBAL TEA

This warming and immune-boosting herbal tea is packed with antioxidants and other beneficial compounds. It can be a go-to drink for those looking to support digestion, promote healing, and aid in weight loss.

INGREDIENTS:

- 2 cups of water
- 1 tablespoon freshly squeezed lemon juice
- 1/2 teaspoon garlic powder
- 1 teaspoon freshly grated ginger
- 1 tablespoon maple syrup or agave syrup (optional for sweetness)

INSTRUCTIONS:

Boil the Water: Start by boiling 2 cups of water in a saucepan or kettle.

Prepare the Ingredients: While the water is heating, prepare your ingredients:

- Juice a fresh lemon to get about 1 tablespoon of juice.
- Grate a small piece of fresh ginger until you have about 1 teaspoon.
- Measure out 1/2 teaspoon of garlic powder (or use a clove of fresh garlic if you prefer a stronger taste).

Combine Ingredients: Once the water is boiling, turn off the heat and let it sit for 1 minute to slightly cool. Then, add the grated ginger and garlic powder to the hot water. Stir well and allow it to steep for about 5-7 minutes.

Strain: If you prefer, strain the tea to remove the grated ginger pieces, or leave them in for added flavor and texture.

Add Lemon Juice: Stir in the freshly squeezed lemon juice right before serving. The lemon adds brightness and a boost of vitamin C to the tea.

Sweeten (Optional): If you like your tea a little sweet, add 1 tablespoon of maple syrup or agave syrup.

Serve: Pour the tea into your favorite mug and enjoy it while warm.

HEALING AND NUTRITION

This simple, natural tea is known to have numerous health benefits, thanks to the combination of its key ingredients. Here's a personal testimony on its effectiveness:

TESTIMONIAL: "*I started drinking this lemon, garlic, and ginger tea when I was feeling under the weather, and it worked wonders in helping me recover quickly. The ginger soothed my stomach, and the garlic helped clear up my congestion, making me feel revitalized within days. After incorporating it into my routine for several weeks, I noticed an improvement in my digestion and metabolism, which helped in my weight loss journey. Drinking this tea 1-2 times a day, especially on an empty stomach, made me feel lighter, less bloated, and full of energy. I highly recommend this blend to anyone looking to improve their overall health naturally.*"

HEALTH BENEFITS:

- **Lemon Juice**: Rich in vitamin C, it boosts the immune system, supports detoxification, and aids in digestion.
- **Garlic Powder**: Known for its antibacterial and anti-inflammatory properties, garlic supports immune health and may improve circulation and metabolism.
- **Ginger**: A powerful anti-inflammatory root that helps with digestion, reduces nausea, and may promote weight loss by increasing fat burning and reducing hunger.

This herbal tea can be a powerful addition to your daily routine for both healing and weight loss support.

VEGAN
Main Dishes

VEGAN CHICKPEA SALAD

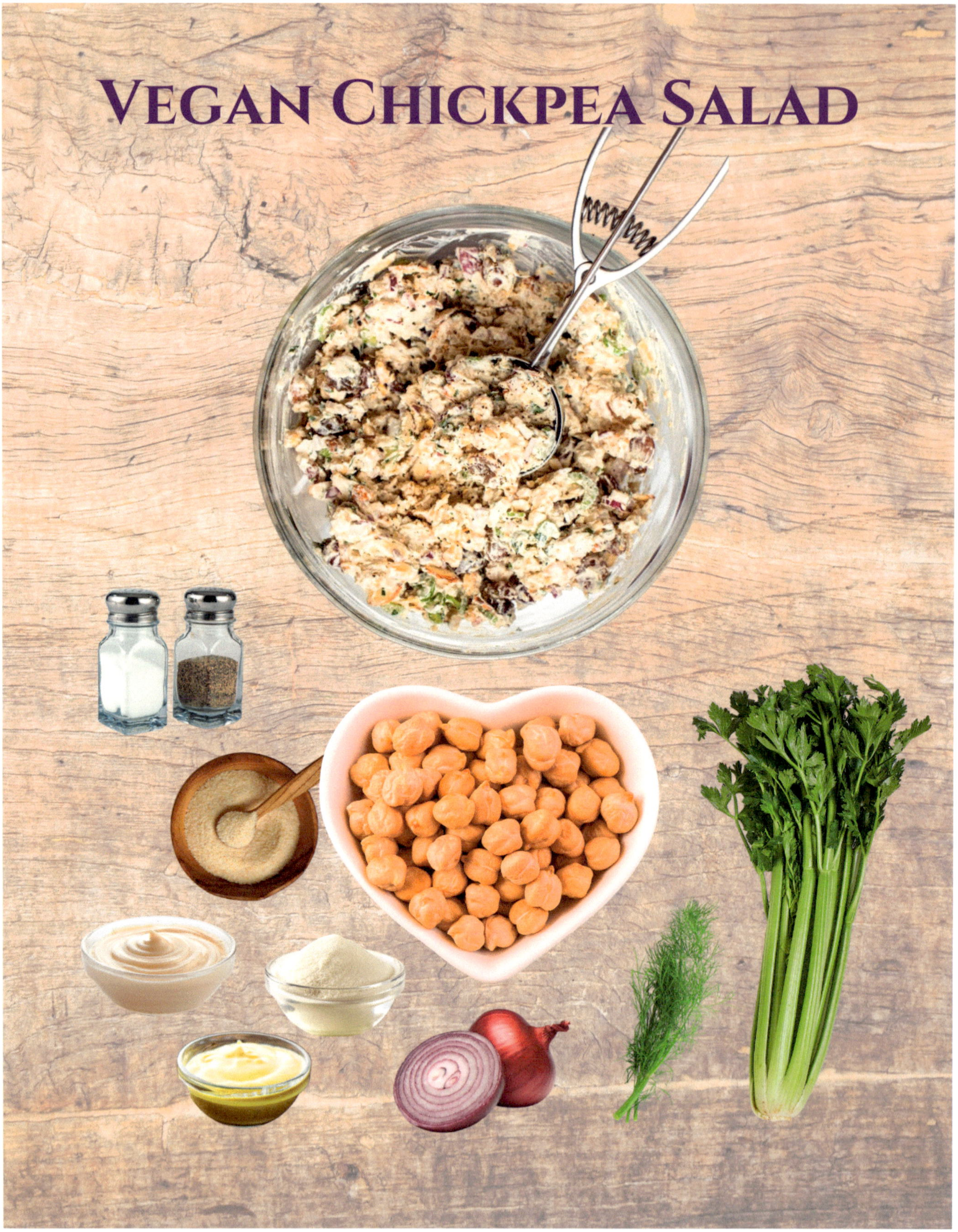

THE SHAWNDA: VEGAN CHICKPEA SALAD

INGREDIENTS:

- 2 cans (15 oz each) chickpeas, drained and rinsed
- 2 stalks of celery, finely chopped
- 1/2 small red onion, finely chopped
- 2-3 tbsp fresh dill, chopped
- 1/2 tsp garlic powder
- 1/2 tsp onion powder
- 1/3 cup of vegan mayonnaise
- 1 tbsp mustard (yellow or Dijon)
- Salt and pepper to taste

INSTRUCTIONS:

Prepare the Chickpeas

Drain and rinse the canned chickpeas under cold water to remove excess sodium. Pat them dry with a paper towel. Place the chickpeas in a large mixing bowl and, using a fork or a potato masher, gently mash about half of them. Leave some chickpeas whole for texture.

Chop the Vegetables

Finely chop the celery and red onion. Make sure the pieces are bite-sized for better distribution in the salad. Add these to the bowl with the chickpeas.

Add Fresh Herbs

Chop the fresh dill and add it to the mixture. The dill adds a fresh, slightly tangy flavor that complements the other ingredients.

Season the Mixture

Add the garlic powder, onion powder, salt, and pepper. These spices give the salad a savory depth and enhance the flavors of the fresh vegetables and herbs.

Incorporate the Dressing

Add the vegan mayonnaise and mustard to the bowl. Mix everything together thoroughly until all ingredients are well coated. The vegan mayo adds creaminess, while the mustard gives a slight kick and tangerines to balance the dish.

Taste and Adjust

Taste the chickpea salad and adjust the seasonings as needed. If you prefer more tang, add a little extra mustard. For a creamier texture, add a bit more vegan mayo. You can also add more dill if you enjoy an extra herbal flavor.

Chill and Serve

Cover the bowl and chill the salad in the refrigerator for at least 30 minutes to allow the flavors to meld together. Serve it on a bed of greens, in a sandwich, or with crackers for a light and satisfying meal.

HEALING AND NUTRITION

The Vegan Chickpea Salad is a powerful addition to any person's health and/or weight loss journey. Packed with protein, fiber, and healthy fats, it is incredibly filling while remaining low in calories. Chickpeas provide plant-based protein and are high in fiber, which supports digestion and helps to maintain a feeling of fullness for longer periods, reducing overeating.

The fresh vegetables, like celery and red onion, offer additional vitamins and minerals while contributing to a crunchy texture, making the salad feel hearty and satisfying. Fresh dill adds not only flavor but also antioxidants that support overall health. By substituting traditional mayonnaise with vegan mayonnaise, the salad becomes heart-healthy, free of cholesterol, and lighter, aiding in weight management.

Incorporating vegan chickpea salad into your diet leads to a noticeable reduction in a person's cravings for processed foods. Which is mainly thanks to its wholesome ingredients and satisfying taste. This can result in him/her finding themselves eating smaller portions and having more energy throughout the day, which can lead to a weight loss of approximately10 pounds over a three-month period. Additionally, the fiber content helps regulate the digestion system, leaving him/her feeling more comfortable and less bloated.

Whether used as a quick lunch, a dinner side, or a snack, this chickpea salad is not only delicious but it is also an empowering addition to any plant-based diet aimed at healing the body and promoting weight loss.

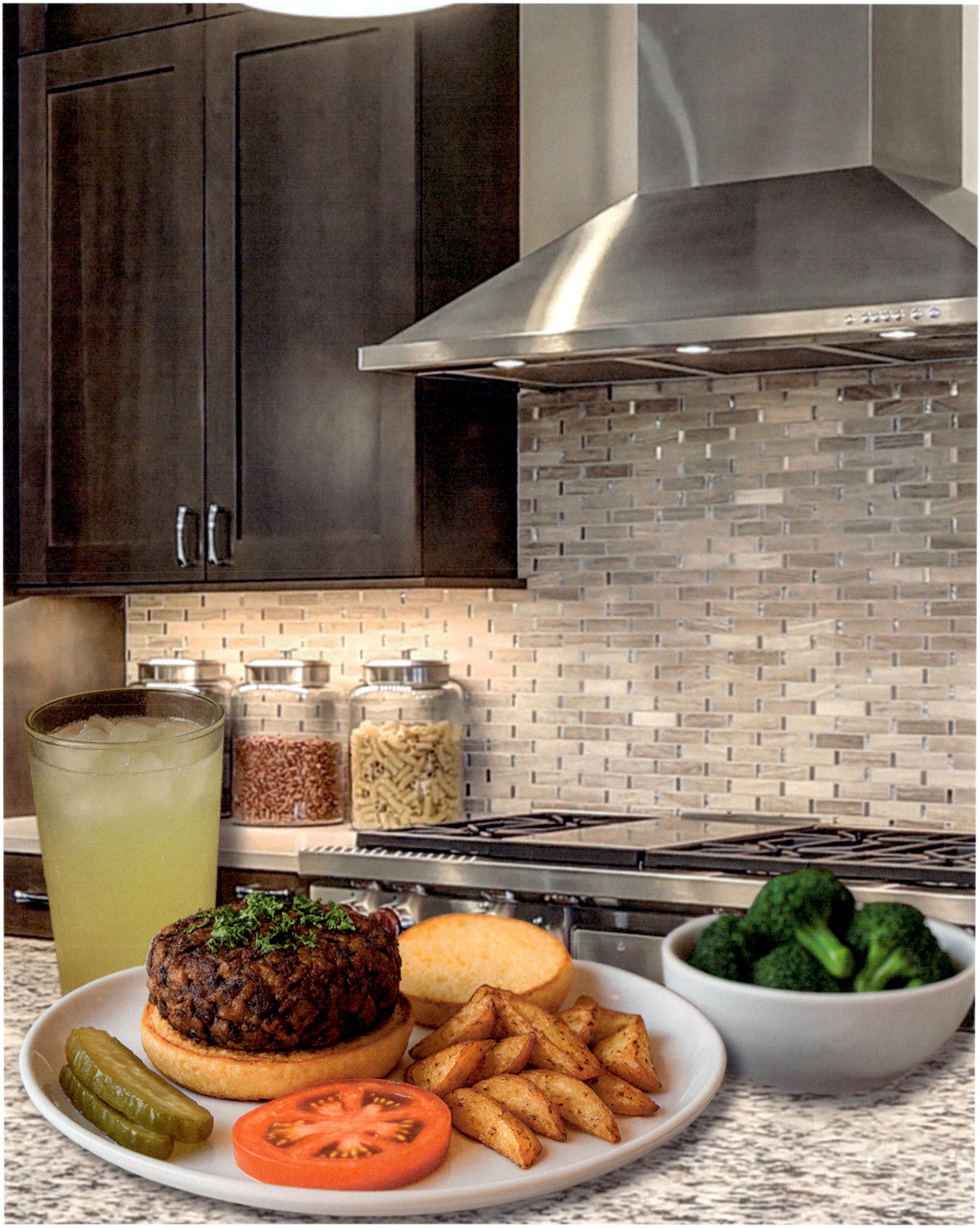

THE CLASSY SIMONE BURGER: VEGAN BLACK BEAN & SHIITAKE MUSHROOM BURGER

INGREDIENTS:

- 2 cups of cooked black beans, drained and rinsed
- 1 cup shiitake mushrooms, finely chopped
- 1 small onion, grated
- 3 cloves garlic, minced
- 1 tablespoon apple cider vinegar
- 1 tablespoon liquid aminos (or soy sauce for a savory flavor)
- 1 teaspoon of Adobo seasoning
- 1 teaspoon smoked paprika
- 1/2 teaspoon black pepper
- 2 tablespoons tomato paste
- 1/4 cup breadcrumbs (optional, for binding)
- 1 tablespoon olive oil (for cooking)

INSTRUCTIONS:

Prepare the Vegetables:

- Finely chop the shiitake mushrooms.
- Grate the onion and mince the garlic.

Cook the Mushrooms and Aromatics:

- Heat a skillet over medium heat and add the olive oil.
- Add the grated onion, garlic, and chopped mushrooms to the skillet.
- Sauté for about 5-7 minutes until the mushrooms release their moisture and the onions become translucent.
- Remove the skillet from the heat and set the mushroom mixture to the side to cool.

Mash the Black Beans:

- In a large mixing bowl, add the drained black beans.
- Using a fork or potato masher, mash the beans until they are mostly smooth, leaving a few whole pieces for texture.

Combine Ingredients:

- Add the cooked mushroom mixture to the mashed black beans.

- Stir in the apple cider vinegar, liquid aminos, adobo seasoning, smoked paprika, black pepper, and tomato paste.
- Mix well until all ingredients are evenly incorporated.
- If the mixture seems too wet, add breadcrumbs one tablespoon at a time until the mixture holds together well.

Form the Patties:

- Divide the mixture into four equal portions and shape each portion into a patty.
- Place the patties on a plate and refrigerate them for at least 30 minutes. This helps them firm up and hold their shape during cooking.

Cook the Patties:

- Heat a skillet or grill pan over medium heat and lightly coat it with a bit of olive oil.
- Cook each patty for about 4-5 minutes per side, or until golden brown and heated through.

Serve:

- Serve the black bean and shiitake mushroom burgers on a bun with your favorite toppings, such as lettuce, tomato, avocado, and a vegan sauce.

HEALING AND NUTRITION

This black bean and shiitake mushroom burger is not only delicious but also highly nutritious, making it a great addition to a healing and weight-loss diet. Black beans are rich in fiber, which helps improve digestion and keep you feeling full longer, reducing the temptation to snack on unhealthy foods. They also provide plant-based protein that supports muscle health and maintains energy levels without the saturated fat found in meat.

Shiitake mushrooms are known for their immune-boosting properties and are low in calories, making them perfect for weight management. They also provide vitamin B, which can improve metabolism and support overall wellness.

This burger contains minimal processed ingredients, and the use of liquid aminos and apple cider vinegar adds a depth of flavor without the need for excessive salt or sugar. The apple cider vinegar is beneficial for balancing pH levels and can aid in weight loss by improving digestion.

Eating this burger regularly as part of a balanced plant-based diet can help reduce inflammation, support digestive health, and contribute to steady weight loss while still enjoying flavorful meals.

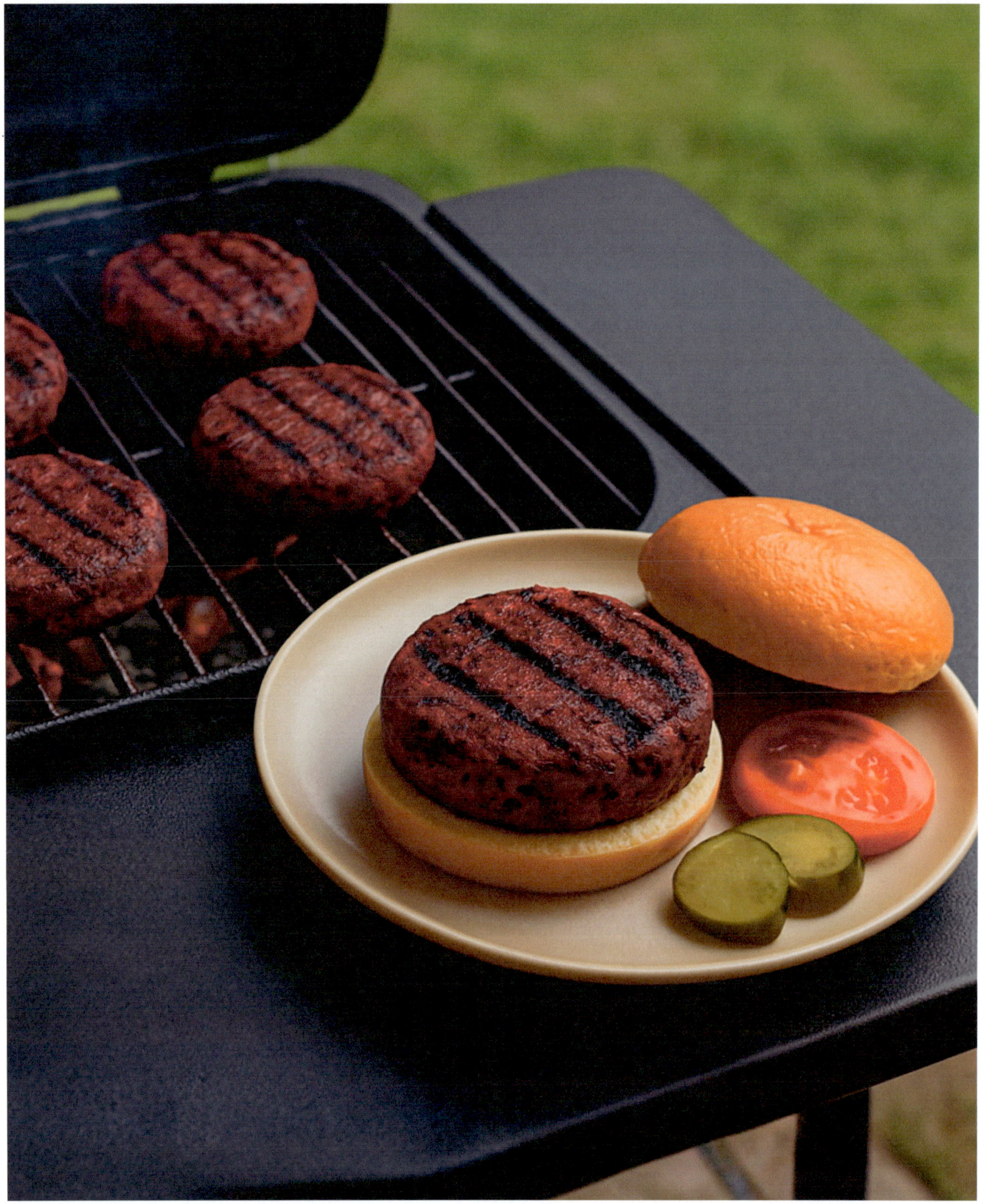

THE MAMA JEAN BURGER: MUSHROOM AND BEET BURGER

INGREDIENTS:

- 2 medium beets, peeled and grated
- 2 large portabella mushrooms, finely chopped
- 1 cup oat flour (you can make your own by blending rolled oats)
- 1 small onion, finely chopped
- 1/4 cup unsweetened applesauce
- 1 teaspoon garlic powder
- 1 teaspoon onion powder
- 1/2 green bell pepper, finely chopped
- 1/2 red bell pepper, finely chopped
- 1/2 yellow bell pepper, finely chopped
- 1/2 orange bell pepper, finely chopped
- 2 Maggi cubes (crushed)
- 1 teaspoon smoked paprika
- 1 tablespoon liquid aminos (or soy sauce)
- 1 tablespoon olive oil (for cooking)

INSTRUCTIONS:

Prepare the Vegetables:

- Peel and grate the beets.
- Finely chop the portabella mushrooms, onion, and the bell peppers.

Cook the Vegetables:

- Heat a large skillet over medium heat and add the olive oil.
- Add the chopped onion, bell peppers, and mushrooms to the skillet.
- Sauté for about 5-7 minutes until the vegetables are softened and the mushrooms release their moisture.
- Add the grated beets to the skillet and cook for an additional 5 minutes.
- Remove the skillet from the heat and let the mixture cool.

Mix the Ingredients:

- In a large mixing bowl, combine the cooled vegetable mixture with the oat flour, applesauce, garlic powder, onion powder, smoked paprika, crushed Maggi cubes, and liquid aminos.
- Mix well until all ingredients are fully incorporated and the mixture holds together.

Form the Patties:

- Divide the mixture into four equal portions and shape each portion into a patty.

- Place the patties on a plate and refrigerate them for at least 30 minutes to help them firm up before cooking.

Cook the Patties:

- Heat a skillet or grill pan over medium heat and lightly grease it with a bit of olive oil.
- Cook each patty for about 4-5 minutes per side, or until they are golden brown and heated through.

Serve:

- Serve the beet and mushroom burgers on a bun with your favorite toppings such as lettuce, tomato, avocado, and a vegan sauce.

HEALING AND NUTRITION

This black mushroom and beet burger is loaded with nutrients that support both healing and weight loss. Beets are rich in antioxidants and nitrates, which help improve blood circulation, reduce inflammation, and boost stamina. They are also low in calories but high in fiber, which helps keep you feeling full longer and supports digestive health.

Portabella mushrooms bring a savory, umami flavor to the burger and provide a good source of B vitamins, which are essential for energy metabolism. Mushrooms are also low in calories and fat, making them ideal for weight management.

The mixture of bell peppers adds a wide range of vitamins, particularly vitamin C, which strengthens the immune system and aids in the absorption of iron from the beets. Using oat flour adds additional fiber and complex carbohydrates, promoting healthy digestion and keeping you satiated.

Incorporating this plant-based burger into a regular diet can support weight loss by providing nutrient-dense, low-calorie ingredients that are filling and satisfying. With no processed or refined ingredients, this burger is ideal for those who want to lose weight while still enjoying delicious, homemade meals that promote healing and overall wellness.

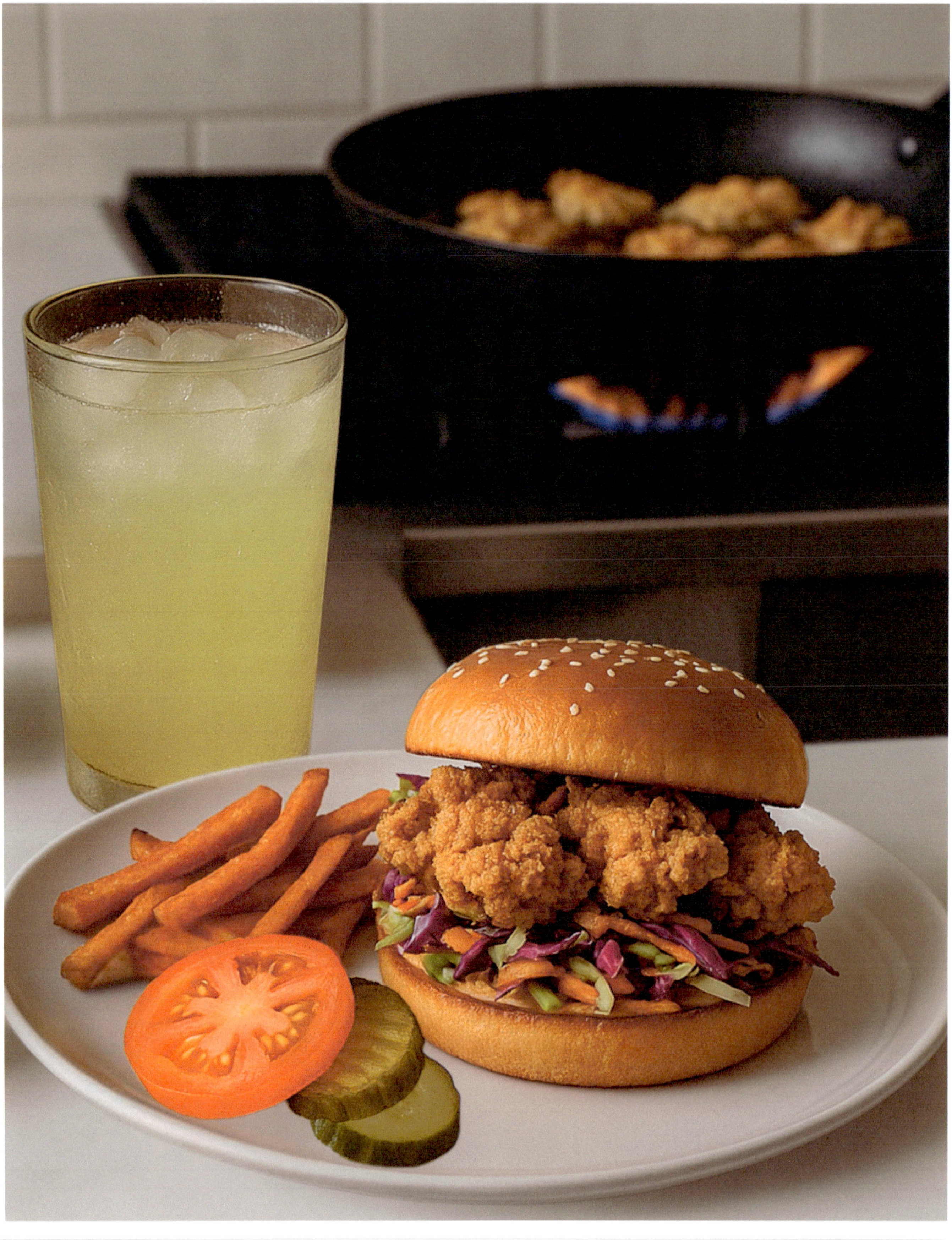

FRIED OYSTER MUSHROOM SANDWICH

INGREDIENTS:

- 2 cups of oyster mushrooms
- 1/2 teaspoon garlic powder
- 1/2 teaspoon onion powder
- 1/2 teaspoon paprika
- 1/2 teaspoon black pepper
- 1 cup coconut milk (unsweetened)
- 1 cup self-rising flour
- 1/2 cup cornmeal
- 1 teaspoon adobo seasoning
- 1 teaspoon paprika
- Grape seed oil (for frying)

MUSHROOM MARINADE:

- 1 teaspoon garlic powder
- 1 teaspoon onion powder
- 1 teaspoon paprika
- 1/2 teaspoon black pepper

For the Sandwich:

- Vegan buns or sandwich bread
- Lettuce leaves
- Sliced tomato
- Vegan mayonnaise (optional)

INSTRUCTIONS:

Marinate the Mushrooms:

- Clean the oyster mushrooms and pat them dry with a paper towel.
- In a bowl, mix 1 teaspoon of garlic powder, 1 teaspoon of onion powder, 1 teaspoon of paprika, and 1/2 teaspoon of black pepper.
- Toss the oyster mushrooms in the spice mixture, ensuring they are evenly coated.
- Let the mushrooms marinate for at least 20-30 minutes to absorb the flavors.

Prepare the Wet and Dry Mixtures:

- In a bowl, pour in the coconut milk and set it aside.
- In a separate bowl, mix the self-rising flour, cornmeal, adobo seasoning, 1 teaspoon of paprika, garlic powder, and onion powder.

Coat the Mushrooms:

- Take each marinated oyster mushroom and dip it into the coconut milk, allowing any excess to drip off.
- Then coat the mushroom in the flour and cornmeal mixture, pressing lightly to ensure a good coating.
- Repeat until all mushrooms are coated.

Fry the Mushrooms:

- Heat grape seed oil in a skillet over medium heat, ensuring there is enough oil to shallow fry the mushrooms.
- Once the oil is hot, carefully place the coated mushrooms in the skillet, frying them in batches to avoid overcrowding.
- Fry each side for 3-4 minutes or until golden brown and crispy.
- Remove the fried mushrooms from the skillet and place them on a plate lined with paper towels to absorb any excess oil.

Assemble the Sandwich:

- Toast the vegan buns or sandwich bread if desired.
- Spread a thin layer of vegan mayonnaise on each side of the bun.
- Place a few lettuce leaves on the bottom bun, add sliced tomatoes, and then add the fried oyster mushrooms on top.
- Top with the other half of the bun.

Serve:

- Serve the sandwich warm with your favorite side, like a green salad or sweet potato fries.

HEALING AND NUTRITION

This vegan fried oyster mushroom sandwich is not only a treat for the taste buds but also a healthy alternative to traditional fried chicken sandwiches. Oyster mushrooms are known for their meaty texture and are packed with nutrients like B vitamins, fiber, and antioxidants, which help reduce inflammation and support the immune system.

The use of coconut milk in this recipe adds healthy fats that can boost metabolism and promote satiety, reducing the desire to snack on unhealthy foods throughout the day. Grape seed oil is chosen for its high smoke point and healthy fatty acids, which are better for the heart compared to traditional frying oils.

Using self-rising flour and cornmeal adds a delicious crispy coating, but the inclusion of spices such as garlic powder, onion powder, and paprika also brings anti-inflammatory properties that aid digestion and metabolism. This sandwich can satisfy cravings for comfort food while still providing a nutritious and plant-based alternative that helps with weight loss and overall well-being.

Incorporating plant-based meals like this fried oyster mushroom sandwich into your diet can significantly support weight loss goals while ensuring you still enjoy delicious, satisfying meals. The fiber, protein, and antioxidants in this recipe make it a filling and nourishing choice, ideal for those looking to reduce calorie intake while enjoying balanced and flavorful dishes.

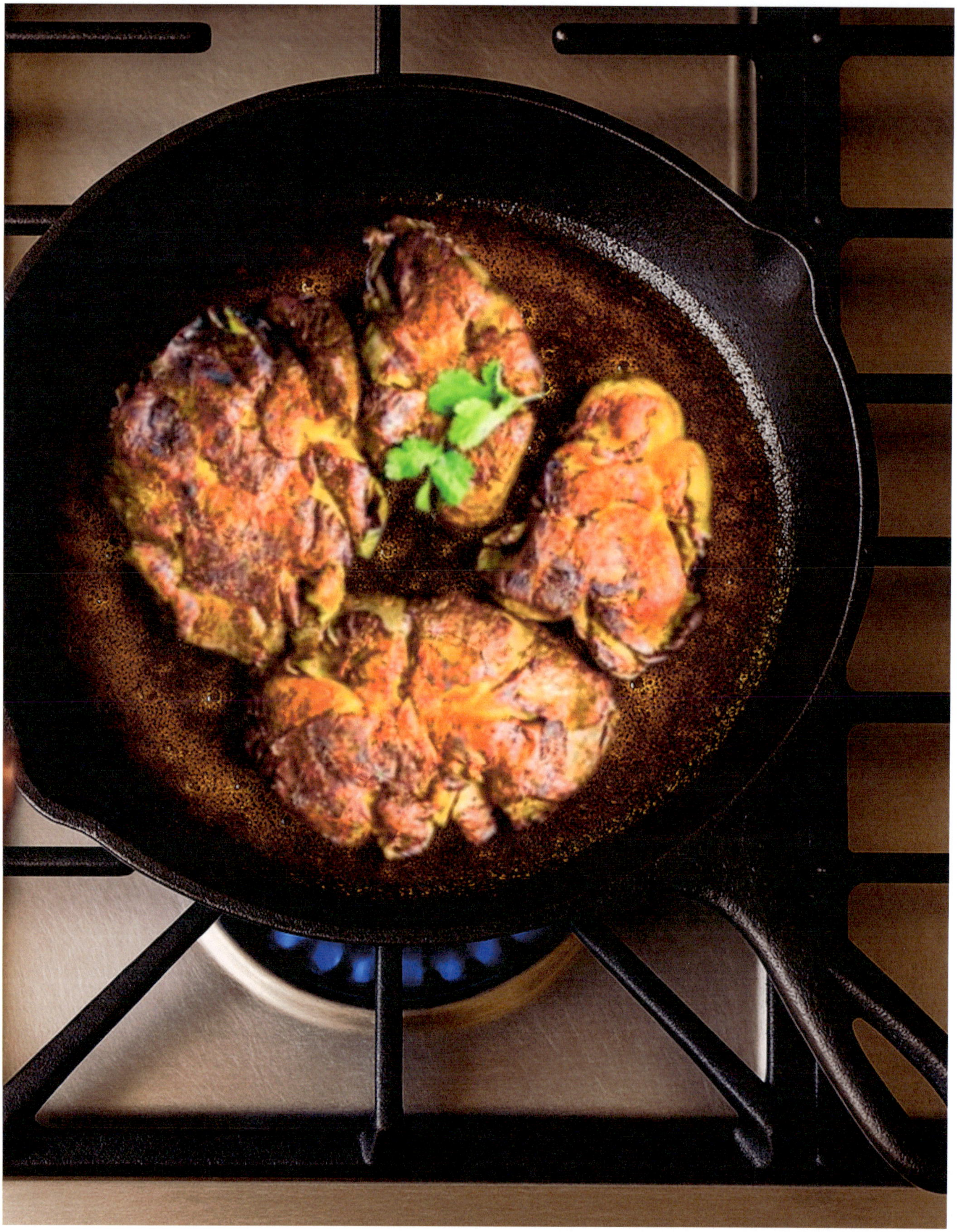

VEGAN BLACK OYSTER MUSHROOM STEAKS

INGREDIENTS:

- 4 large oyster mushroom clusters
- 1 teaspoon garlic powder
- 1 teaspoon onion powder
- 1 teaspoon smoked paprika
- 1/2 teaspoon black pepper
- 1 teaspoon adobo seasoning
- 1 cup coconut milk (unsweetened)
- 1 cup self-rising flour
- 1/2 cup cornmeal
- 2 tablespoons grape seed oil (for searing)

INSTRUCTIONS:

Prepare the Mushrooms:

- Clean the oyster mushrooms and trim the ends if necessary. Gently press them to flatten slightly so that they resemble steaks.

Marinate the Mushrooms:

- In a bowl, combine the garlic powder, onion powder, smoked paprika, black pepper, and adobo seasoning.
- Rub the spice mixture evenly over the mushrooms, ensuring they are well coated.
- Let the mushrooms marinate for at least 20-30 minutes to allow the flavors to penetrate.

Prepare the Wet and Dry Coatings:

- In a bowl, add coconut milk.
- In a separate bowl, mix the self-rising flour and cornmeal together.

Coat the Mushrooms:

- Take each marinated oyster mushroom cluster and dip it into the coconut milk, making sure it is fully coated.
- Then dredge the mushroom cluster in the flour and cornmeal mixture, pressing gently to ensure the coating sticks.
- Repeat with all mushroom clusters.

Sear the Mushroom Steaks:

- Heat a large skillet over medium-high heat and add the grape seed oil.
- Once the oil is hot, add the coated oyster mushroom clusters to the skillet.
- Sear each side for about 3-4 minutes, or until golden brown and crispy.
- Remove from the skillet and place on a plate lined with paper towels to absorb any excess oil.

Serve:

- Serve the oyster mushroom steaks hot, with your favorite sides such as mashed potatoes, roasted vegetables, or a fresh green salad.

HEALING AND NUTRITION

This vegan oyster mushroom steak is an excellent dish for anyone looking to improve their health and support weight loss. Oyster mushrooms have a meaty texture, making them a perfect substitute for traditional meat, and are loaded with beneficial nutrients such as B vitamins, selenium, and fiber, which help boost immunity and promote healthy digestion.

Coconut milk is used in this recipe for its healthy fats, which help increase satiety and reduce overeating. The spices, including paprika, garlic powder, and onion powder, not only add delicious flavor but also provide antioxidants that reduce inflammation and support metabolism.

The self-rising flour and cornmeal create a crispy coating that gives the oyster mushrooms a satisfying texture without adding too many calories. Cornmeal adds fiber and gives a wholesome taste, while grape seed oil is a healthier choice for frying due to its high smoke point and heart-healthy fats.

Using plant-based alternatives such as these mushroom steaks can help reduce calorie intake while still providing a satisfying, hearty meal. The combination of fiber, healthy fats, and antioxidants supports a balanced diet that aids in weight loss and overall wellness. Regularly incorporating dishes like this into your diet can help curb meat cravings and promote a healthier, more sustainable lifestyle without compromising on flavor.

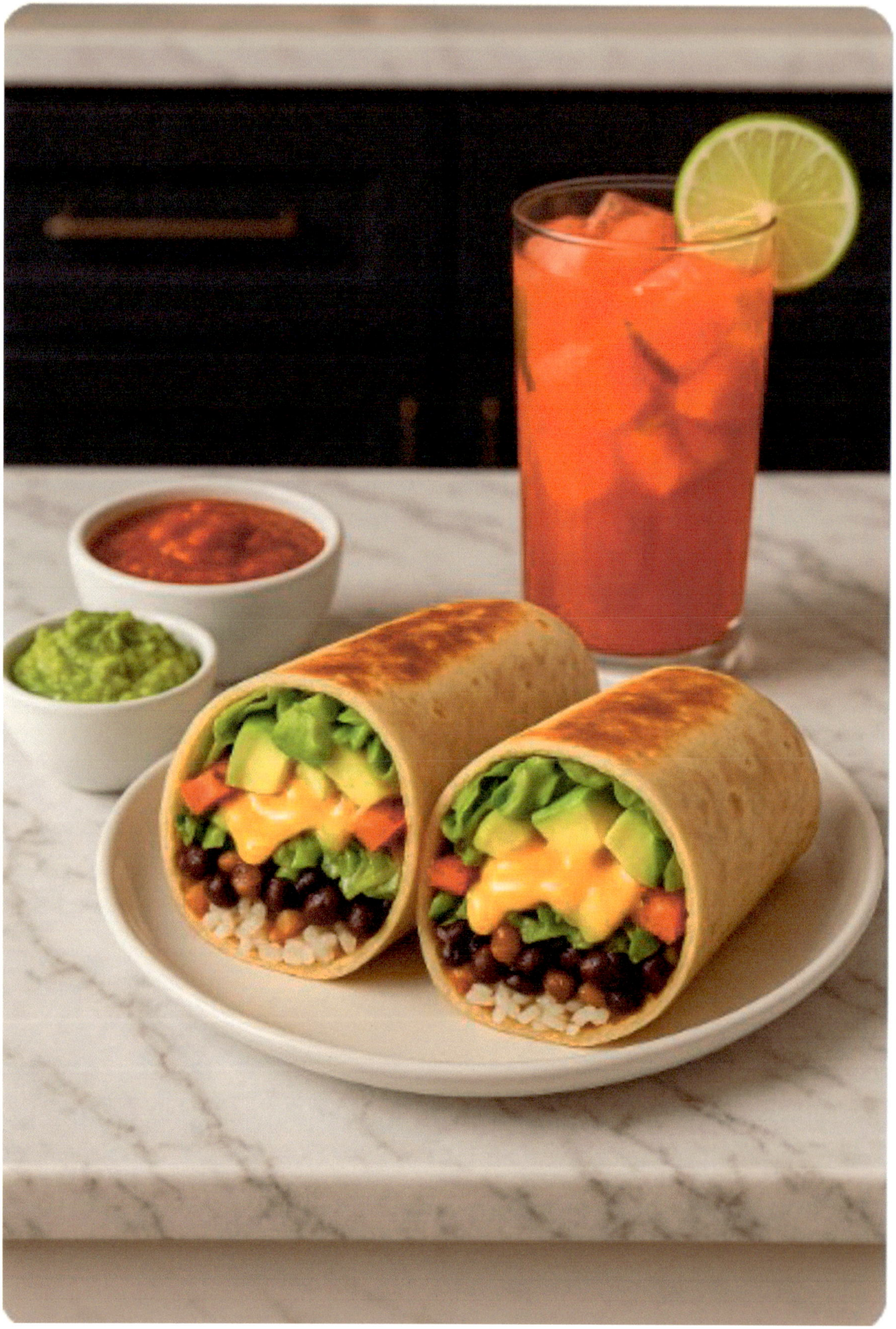

VEGAN BLACK BEAN BURRITO

INGREDIENTS:

- 1 can (15 oz) black beans, drained and rinsed
- 1 cup cooked brown or white rice
- 1 cup diced tomatoes
- 1 cup shredded lettuce
- 1 ripe avocado, sliced
- 1/2 cup vegan cheese (shredded)
- 4 large corn tortilla wraps

INSTRUCTIONS:

Prepare the Ingredients:

- Cook the brown or white rice according to the package instructions. If using leftovers, warm the rice slightly in a skillet or microwave.
- Drain and rinse the black beans and set them aside.
- Dice the tomatoes, shred the lettuce, and slice the avocado.

Warm the Tortilla Wraps:

- In a skillet over medium heat, warm each tortilla wrap for about 15-20 seconds on each side, until pliable.

Assemble the Burritos:

- Place a warmed tortilla wrap on a clean surface.
- Start by adding a layer of cooked rice in the center of the tortilla, leaving some space around the edges.
- Add a generous scoop of black beans on top of the rice.
- Sprinkle diced tomatoes over the beans, followed by shredded lettuce.
- Add a few slices of avocado.
- Sprinkle with vegan cheese.
- Be careful not to overfill, as it will make wrapping difficult.

Wrap the Burritos:

- Fold the sides of the tortilla over the filling, then roll it up from the bottom to the top, tucking in the sides as you go, to form a burrito.
- Repeat the process with the remaining tortillas and ingredients.

Serve:

- Serve the burritos as is or toast them lightly in a skillet for a crispy exterior.
- Slice in half and serve with your favorite salsa or guacamole on the side.

HEALING AND NUTRITION:

This vegan black bean burrito is packed with nutrients that support both healing and weight loss. Black beans are a great source of plant-based protein and fiber, which help you stay full longer and promote healthy digestion, both of which are important for weight management. They also contain antioxidants and phytonutrients that support heart health and reduce inflammation.

Brown or white rice provides a good source of energy and helps make the burrito more satisfying. Brown rice is rich in fiber, which keeps your blood sugar levels stable and further supports digestive health. Avocado adds healthy fats, which help absorb fat-soluble vitamins and promote satiety, reducing the urge to overeat.

Fresh vegetables, such as tomatoes and lettuce, add essential vitamins and minerals to this burrito, while the corn tortilla wrap keeps the dish gluten-free and easier on digestion. Vegan cheese adds a touch of indulgence without the saturated fat found in dairy cheese.

Incorporating plant-based meals like this black bean burrito into your diet can help you reach your weight loss goals in a balanced way. It provides ample fiber, protein, and healthy fats that keep you satisfied while also offering a nutrient-dense, low-calorie meal. This burrito is a perfect example of how to enjoy a delicious, filling meal while supporting your overall health and wellness journey.

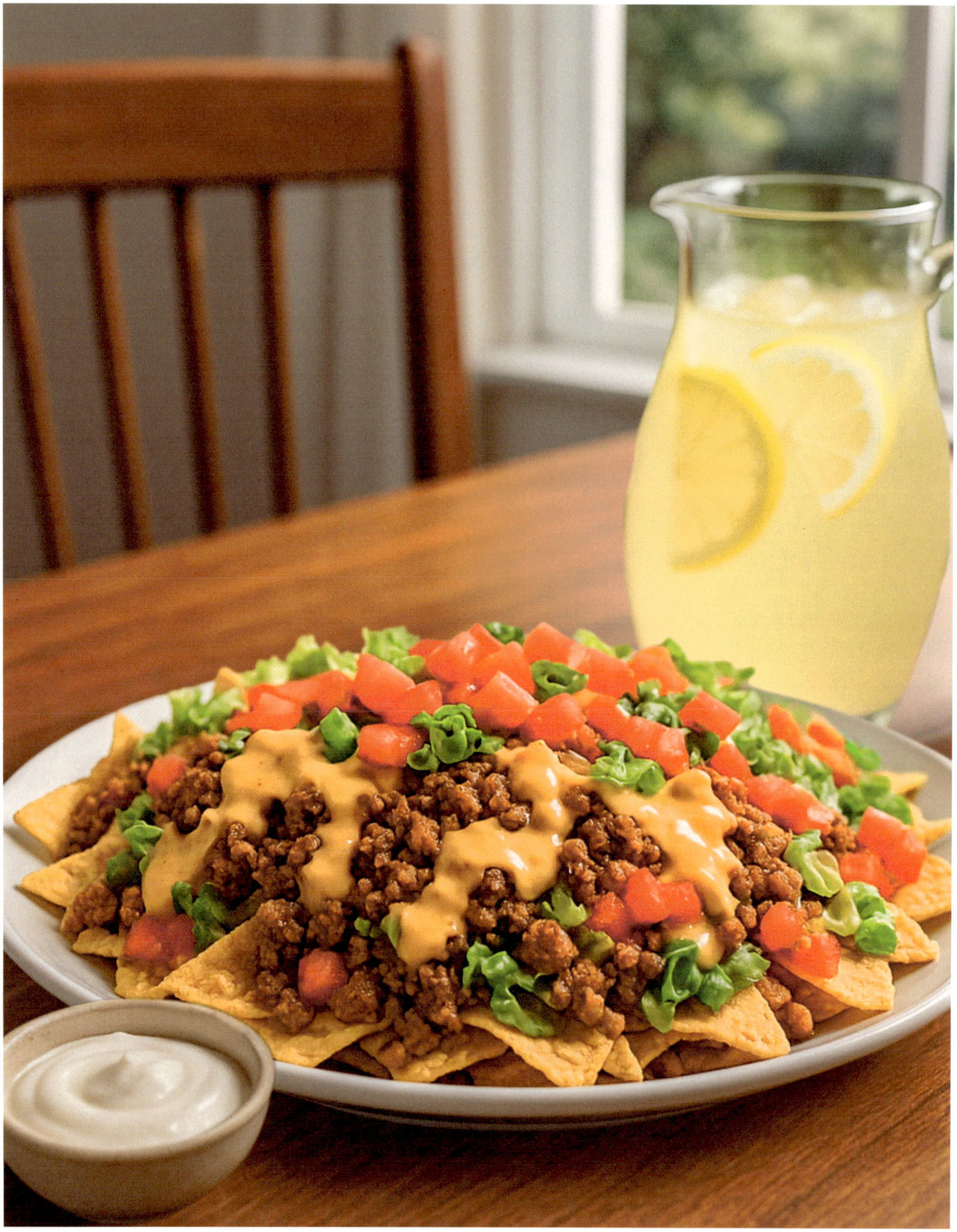

THE VT: VEGAN NACHOS AND CHEESE

INGREDIENTS:

For the Topping:

- 1 cup walnuts
- 1 cup mushrooms, finely chopped
- 1/2 green bell pepper, finely chopped
- 1/2 red bell pepper, finely chopped
- 1 teaspoon garlic powder
- 1 teaspoon onion powder
- 1 teaspoon smoked paprika
- 1 tablespoon olive oil
- 1 cup shredded lettuce
- 1 cup diced tomatoes
- Sliced jalapeño peppers (optional)

For the Vegan Cheese Sauce:

- 1 cup cashews (soaked in hot water for at least 30 minutes)
- 1/4 cup coconut milk (unsweetened)
- 2 tablespoons nutritional yeast
- 1/2 teaspoon onion powder
- 1/2 teaspoon garlic powder
- 1/4 teaspoon smoked paprika
- 1-2 tablespoons water (to adjust consistency)

For the Nachos:

- 1 bag corn chips

INSTRUCTIONS:

Prepare the Walnut-Mushroom Topping:

- In a food processor, pulse the walnuts until they resemble ground meat.
- Heat a skillet over medium heat and add the olive oil.
- Add the chopped mushrooms, green bell pepper, and red bell pepper. Sauté for about 5-7 minutes until the vegetables are softened.
- Add the walnuts to the skillet along with the garlic powder, onion powder, and smoked paprika.
- Stir well and cook for another 5-7 minutes until the mixture is well combined and heated through, and set the mixture to the side.

Prepare the Vegan Cheese Sauce:

- Drain and rinse the soaked cashews.
- In a blender, combine the cashews, coconut milk, nutritional yeast, garlic powder, onion powder, and smoked paprika.
- Blend until smooth and creamy. Add 1-2 tablespoons of water if needed to achieve a smooth cheese-like consistency.

Assemble the Nachos:

- Spread a generous layer of corn chips on a large serving platter or baking tray.
- Evenly distribute the walnut-mushroom topping over the corn chips.
- Drizzle the vegan cheese sauce generously over the toppings.
- Add shredded lettuce, diced tomatoes, and sliced jalapeño peppers (if using) for extra flavor and crunch.

Serve:

- Serve the nachos immediately as is, or warm them in the oven at 350°F (175°C) for about 10 minutes for a warm and slightly melted experience.
- Enjoy with extra cheese sauce or salsa on the side for dipping.

HEALING AND NUTRITION

This vegan nachos and cheese recipe is not only delicious but also provides various nutrients that support weight loss and overall healing. Walnuts are rich in omega-3 fatty acids and protein, which are beneficial for heart health and help reduce inflammation. The combination of walnuts and mushrooms creates a hearty and satisfying topping that makes these nachos filling and nutritious.

Mushrooms are low in calories and are an excellent source of vitamins and antioxidants, which support immune health. The bell peppers add a good dose of vitamin C, which helps boost immunity, and fiber, which helps keep you full.

The vegan cheese sauce made from cashews is creamy and indulgent, without the cholesterol found in dairy cheese. Cashews provide healthy fats, which are important for brain health and help with satiety, reducing overeating. Nutritional yeast adds a cheesy flavor while providing a source of B vitamins that support energy production and metabolism.

Using corn chips and topping them with fresh vegetables like lettuce, tomatoes, and optional jalapeño peppers ensures the dish stays vibrant and refreshing. Jalapeños contain capsaicin, which may boost metabolism and help in weight loss.

By replacing traditional nacho cheese and meat with healthier, plant-based alternatives, you can enjoy a satisfying dish without unnecessary calories, saturated fats, and cholesterol. These nachos are a perfect example of how you can still enjoy comfort food while making choices that support your health and weight loss goals. They provide a good balance of protein, fiber, and healthy fats, making them a great addition to a healthy diet.

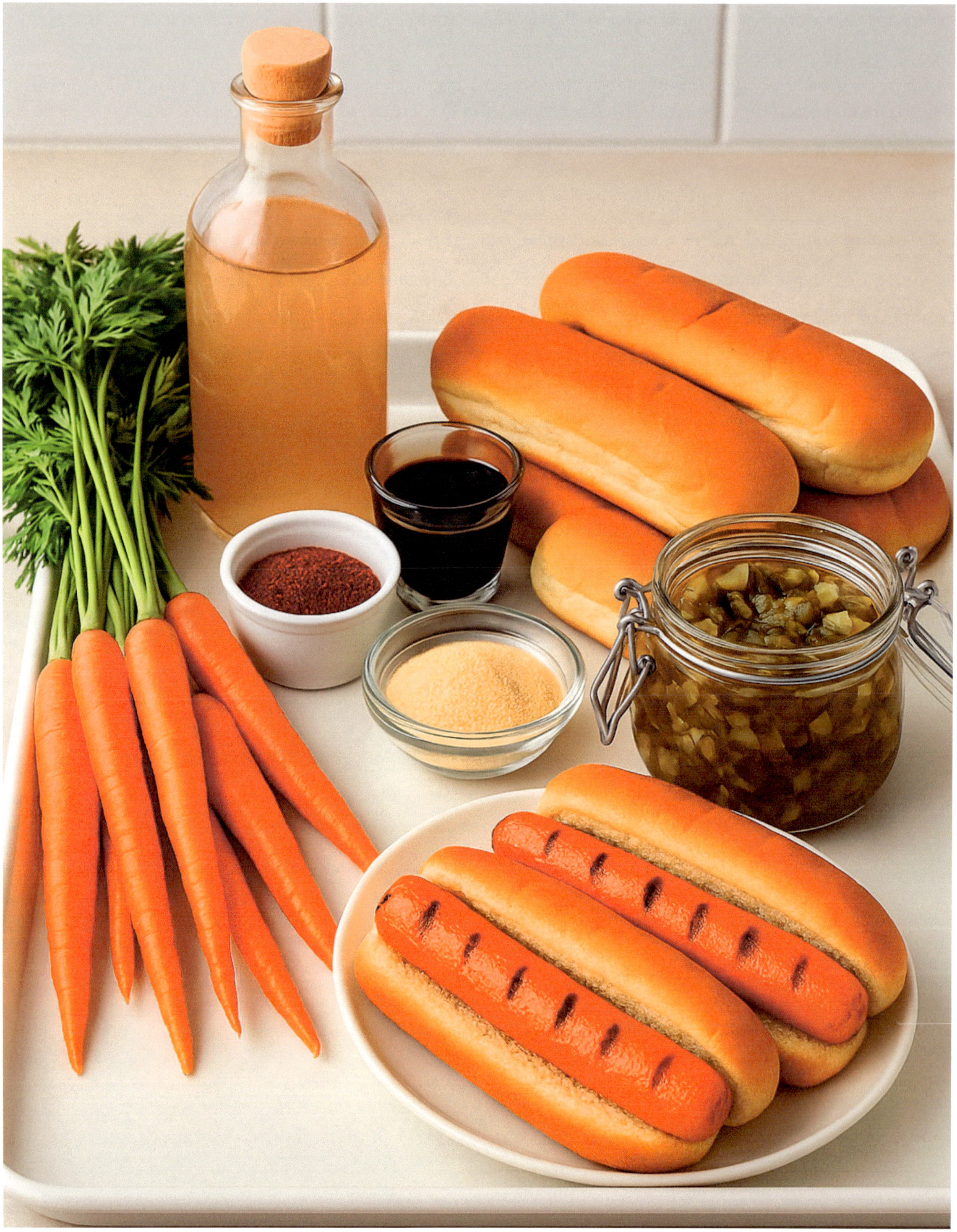

VEGAN CARROT DOGS

INGREDIENTS:

- 6 large carrots (peeled, trimmed to fit into hot dog buns)
- 2 cloves garlic, minced
- 1 small onion, finely chopped
- 1 teaspoon mixed herb seasonings (such as thyme, rosemary, and oregano)
- 1 teaspoon smoked paprika
- 3 cups water

INSTRUCTIONS:

Prepare the Carrots:

- Peel the carrots and trim the ends so that they fit into a hot dog bun.
- Boil 3 cups of water in a medium-sized pot. Add the peeled and trimmed carrots.
- Cook the carrots for about 10-15 minutes, or until they are fork-tender but not too soft. They should have a texture similar to a hot dog.

Prepare the Marinade:

- In a small saucepan, heat a little water and sauté the minced garlic and chopped onion for about 3-4 minutes, or until softened and aromatic.
- Add smoked paprika, herb seasonings, and 1/4 cup of water to the saucepan. Mix well and allow to simmer for another 2 minutes.

Marinate the Carrots:

- Place the boiled carrots in a shallow dish or container.
- Pour the marinade over the carrots, making sure they are fully coated.
- Cover the container and refrigerate for at least 4 hours, or ideally overnight, for maximum flavor.

Cook the Carrot Dogs:

- Preheat a skillet or grill over medium heat.
- Remove the carrots from the marinade and grill them for about 5-7 minutes, rotating to ensure even cooking and slight charring.

Serve:

- Place the cooked carrot dogs into hot dog buns and top with your favorite toppings, such as mustard, ketchup, chopped onions, or pickles.
- Serve immediately and enjoy!

HEALING AND NUTRITION:

These vegan carrot dogs are a great low-calorie and nutrient-dense alternative to traditional hot dogs. Carrots are rich in beta-carotene, an antioxidant that supports eye health, immune function, and skin health. They are also a good source of dietary fiber, which aids digestion and helps you stay full longer, making them an ideal food for weight loss.

The herb seasonings and smoked paprika add layers of flavor without any added fat or cholesterol. This helps keep the dish light, while the garlic and onion provide additional immune-boosting properties and natural anti-inflammatory effects.

Using carrot dogs instead of processed meat hot dogs can significantly reduce your intake of unhealthy fats, sodium, and preservatives, which are common in traditional hot dogs. These carrot dogs provide a nutrient-rich option that can satisfy cravings while supporting healing and weight loss. This plant-based twist on a classic comfort food helps to eliminate the empty calories and harmful substances found in conventional hot dogs, promoting a more balanced and health-conscious way of eating.

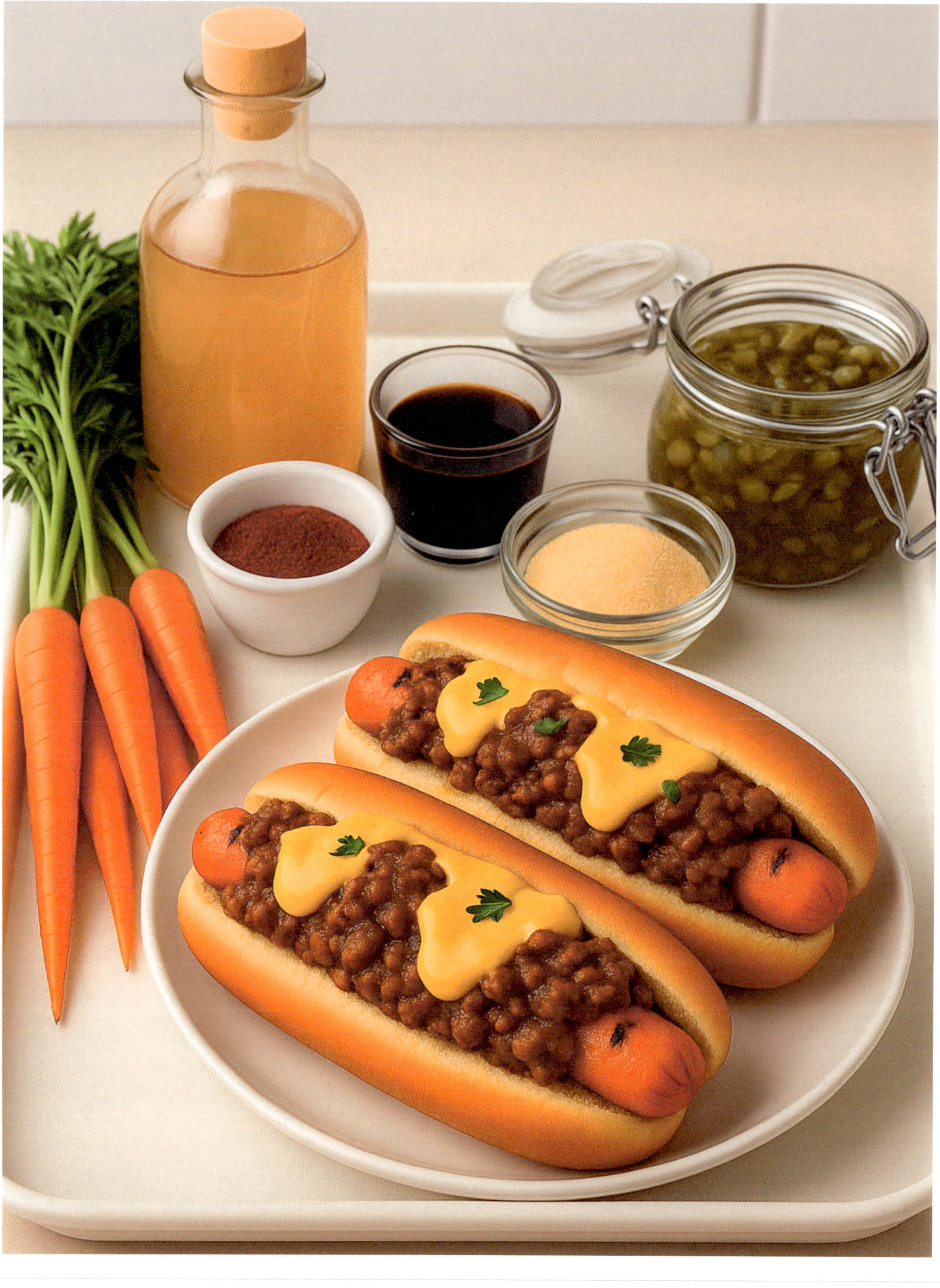

THE DARYL DOG: VEGAN CHILI CHEESE CARROT DOGS

INGREDIENTS:

For the Carrot Dogs:

- 6 large carrots (peeled and trimmed to fit into hot dog buns)
- 1 cup walnuts (finely chopped)
- 1 cup mushrooms (finely chopped)
- 1-2 chili peppers (finely chopped, adjust to taste)
- 3 cloves garlic (minced)
- Hot dog buns
- 1 teaspoon mixed herb seasonings (e.g., thyme, oregano, basil)
- 1 teaspoon smoked paprika
- 1 small onion (finely chopped)
- Chopped green onions or cilantro (optional, for garnish)
- Salt and pepper to taste
- 2 cups water

For the Vegan Cheese Sauce:

- 1 cup raw cashews (soaked in hot water for at least 30 minutes)
- 1/4 cup nutritional yeast
- 1/2 teaspoon garlic powder
- 1/2 teaspoon onion powder
- 1/2 teaspoon smoked paprika
- 1/4 cup water (more as needed)

INSTRUCTIONS:

Prepare the Carrots:

- Peel the carrots and trim the ends so they fit into hot dog buns.
- Boil 2 cups of water in a medium-sized pot. Add the peeled and trimmed carrots.
- Cook the carrots for about 10-15 minutes, or until they are fork-tender but still firm enough to hold their shape. Drain and set aside.

Make the Walnut-Mushroom Filling:

- In a skillet over medium heat, add a little water (or olive oil if desired) and sauté the chopped onion and garlic until they become translucent (about 3-4 minutes).

- Add the chopped mushrooms, walnuts, chopped chili peppers, smoked paprika, and herb seasonings. Sauté for another 5-7 minutes, until the mushrooms are cooked down and the mixture is fragrant.
- Season with salt and pepper to taste. Remove from heat and set aside.

Prepare the Vegan Cheese Sauce:

- Drain and rinse the soaked cashews.
- In a blender, combine the cashews, nutritional yeast, garlic powder, onion powder, smoked paprika, and 1/4 cup of water.
- Blend until smooth and creamy, adding more water as necessary to reach a cheese-like consistency.

Assemble the Chili Cheese Carrot Dogs:

- Place a boiled carrot in a hot dog bun.
- Spoon the walnut-mushroom filling generously over the carrot.
- Drizzle the vegan cheese sauce on top.
- Optionally, garnish with chopped green onions or cilantro.

Serve:

- Serve the chili cheese carrot dogs immediately, with extra cheese sauce on the side if desired.

HEALING AND NUTRITION

These vegan chili cheese carrot dogs are a nutritious and filling option for anyone looking to enjoy comfort food while supporting their health goals.

Carrots are packed with vitamins A and C, as well as dietary fiber, which aids in digestion and helps maintain a healthy weight. They provide natural sweetness and a satisfying crunch, making them a great low-calorie alternative to traditional hot dogs.

Walnuts are an excellent source of healthy fats and protein, promoting heart health and reducing inflammation. They help to keep you satiated, making it easier to control cravings and reduce overall calorie intake.

Mushrooms are low in calories

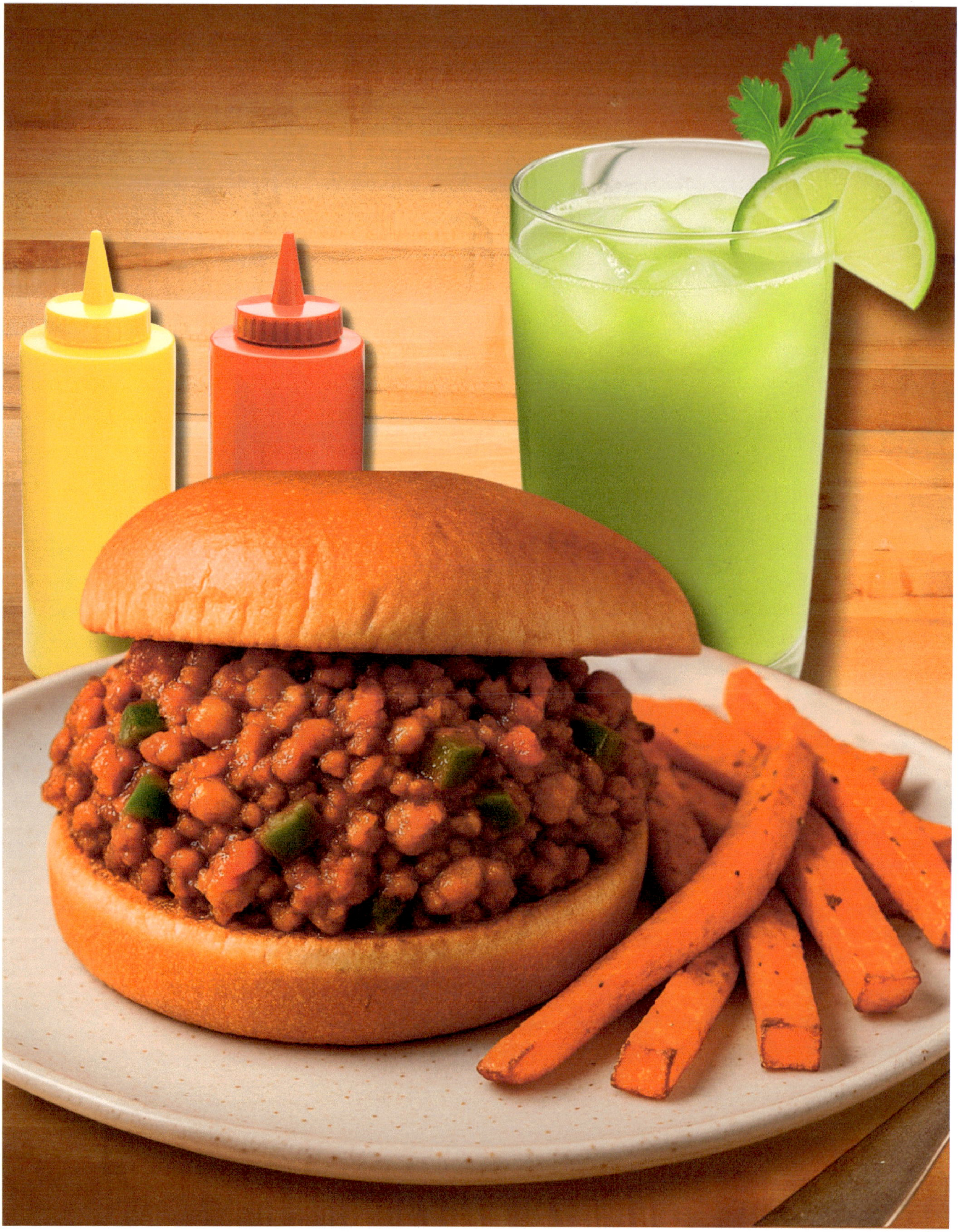

THE SUAVEY: VEGAN WALNUT SLOPPY JOE

This vegan walnut sloppy joe recipe is a satisfying, protein-rich twist on the classic dish, using walnuts instead of meat. It is seasoned with flavorful spices like paprika, garlic powder, and onion powder, and features green pepper and tomato paste to create a hearty, nutritious meal. Walnuts add a delicious crunch and provide healthy fats that support weight loss and overall wellness.

INGREDIENTS:

- 1 cup raw walnuts
- 2 tablespoons tomato paste
- 1/2 teaspoon garlic powder
- 1/2 teaspoon onion powder
- 1/4 teaspoon black pepper (or to taste)
- 1/2 teaspoon smoked paprika (or regular paprika)
- Vegan buns or whole wheat buns for serving
- Salt to taste
- 1 small green pepper, diced
- 1 small onion, diced (optional for extra flavor)
- 1 tablespoon olive oil or grapeseed oil (optional for sautéing)
- 1/2 cup water or vegetable broth (for moisture)
- 2 tablespoons soy sauce or tamari (optional, for added umami flavor)

INSTRUCTIONS:

Prepare the Walnuts:

- Start by soaking the walnuts in hot water for about 10-15 minutes to soften them. Drain and rinse well.
- After soaking, pulse the walnuts in a food processor until they are finely chopped, resembling ground meat. Be careful not to over-process them into a paste.

Sauté the Vegetables (Optional):

- In a medium-sized skillet, heat 1 tablespoon of oil over medium heat. Add the diced green pepper (and onion if using), and sauté for about 4-5 minutes until they soften and become fragrant. If you prefer an oil-free version, you can skip this step and add the veggies directly in the next step with water or broth.

Cook the Walnut Mixture:

- Add the chopped walnuts to the skillet with the softened green pepper.
- Stir in the tomato paste, garlic powder, onion powder, smoked paprika, black pepper, and a pinch of salt.
- Pour in the water or vegetable broth and stir to combine everything evenly. If you are using soy sauce or tamari for extra flavor, add that now as well.

Simmer:

- Reduce the heat to low and let the mixture simmer for 10-15 minutes, stirring occasionally. The walnuts should absorb the flavors, and the sauce will thicken.
- Taste and adjust seasoning, adding more salt, black pepper, or paprika as needed.

Assemble the Sloppy Joes:

- Toast your vegan buns if desired and spoon the walnut sloppy joe mixture generously onto each bun.
- Serve with a side salad or sweet potato fries for a balanced meal.

Enjoy:

- Serve hot and enjoy the flavorful, hearty texture of this plant-based sloppy joe.

HEALING AND NUTRITION

TESTIMONIAL: "*This walnut sloppy joe recipe was a game changer for me! I was looking for plant-based alternatives that could satisfy my cravings for comfort food while still being healthy, and this dish fits the bill perfectly. The walnuts provide a great source of healthy fats and protein, which kept me feeling full and energized for hours. I noticed that after incorporating this recipe into my meal rotation, I was able to manage my appetite better and cut down on unhealthy snacking. It's amazing how something this delicious can also support my weight loss journey. The combination of tomato paste, garlic powder, and paprika gave the dish a rich, smoky flavor that made it taste just like the traditional sloppy joes I used to love, but without the heaviness!*"

Health Benefits:

- **Walnuts**: Rich in omega-3 fatty acids, protein, and fiber, walnuts support heart health, reduce inflammation, and help keep you full longer, aiding in weight management.
- **Tomato Paste**: A concentrated source of lycopene, an antioxidant that supports heart health and helps fight inflammation.
- **Garlic and Onion Powder**: Provide anti-inflammatory and immune-boosting benefits while adding savory flavor.
- **Green Pepper**: High in vitamins A and C, green peppers support immune health and provide a low-calorie way to add bulk and nutrition to the meal.
- **Paprika**: Adds a rich, smoky flavor and contains antioxidants that support overall health.

This vegan walnut sloppy joe is not only delicious but also packed with nutrients that promote healing and support weight loss by keeping you full and satisfied!

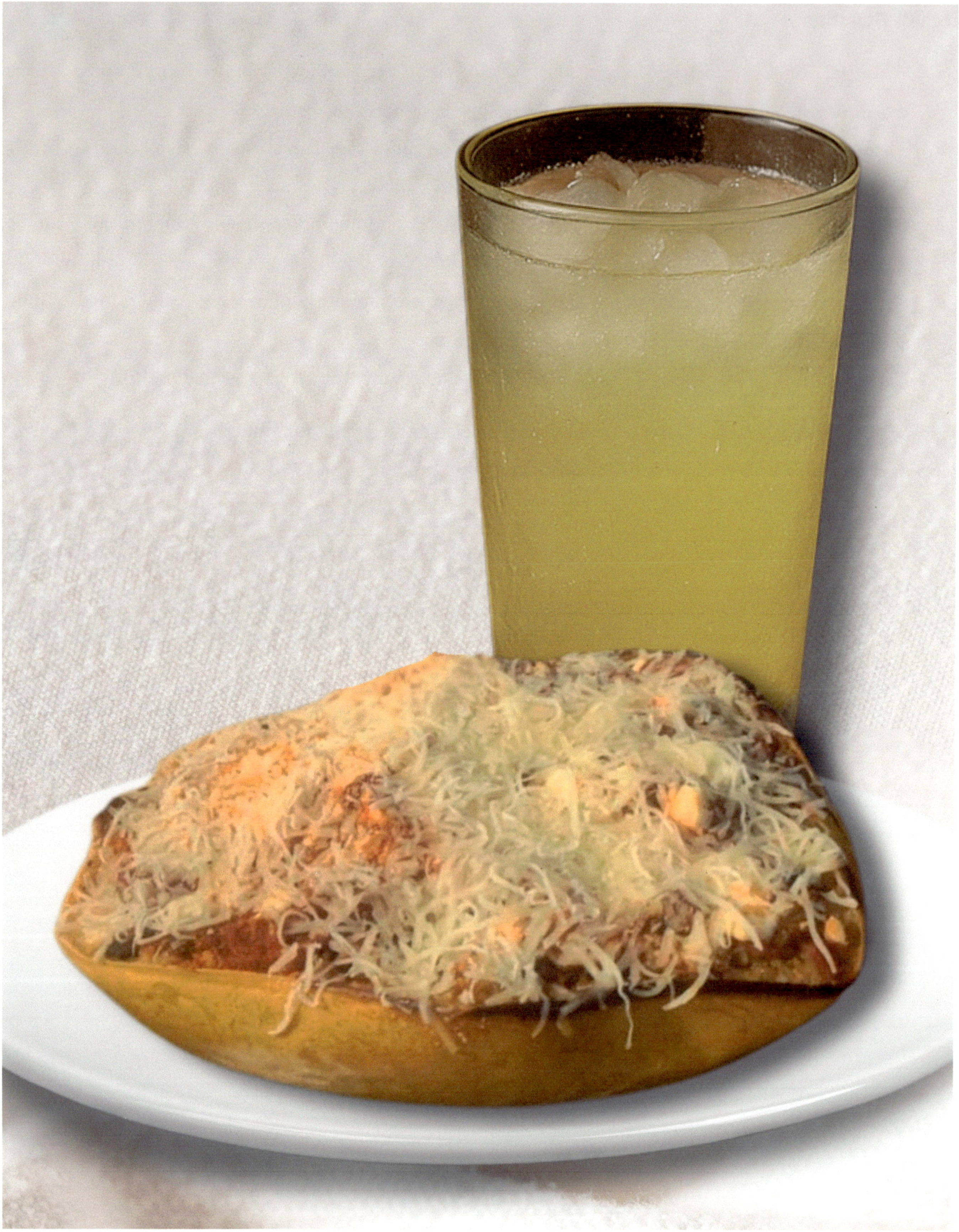

THE TIFF: VEGAN BAKED SPAGHETTI SQUASH WITH VEGAN CHEESE

INGREDIENTS:

- 1 large spaghetti squash
- 1 cup shredded vegan cheese (mozzarella or cheddar-style)
- 1/4 cup vegan parmesan cheese
- 1 teaspoon garlic powder
- 1 tablespoon dried oregano
- 1 teaspoon onion powder
- 2 tablespoons olive oil or vegan butter
- Salt and black pepper to taste
- 1 tablespoon dried parsley

INSTRUCTIONS:

Step 1: Prepare the Spaghetti Squash

1. **Preheat the oven** to 400°F (200°C). Line a baking sheet with parchment paper.
2. **Cut the spaghetti squash** in half lengthwise and scoop out the seeds using a spoon.
3. **Drizzle the squash** with olive oil or vegan butter and sprinkle with a pinch of salt and black pepper.
4. **Place the squash halves** cut-side down on the baking sheet and roast in the preheated oven for 35-45 minutes, or until the squash is tender and can easily be scraped into spaghetti-like strands with a fork.

Step 2: Mix the Cheese and Seasoning

1. While the squash is baking, prepare the cheese mixture. In a small bowl, combine the shredded vegan cheese, garlic powder, onion powder, dried oregano, dried parsley, and half of the vegan parmesan cheese.
2. Mix everything well to evenly distribute the seasonings throughout the cheese.

Step 3: Shred the Spaghetti Squash

1. Once the spaghetti squash is cooked, remove it from the oven and let it cool slightly for about 5-10 minutes.
2. Using a fork, gently scrape the inside of the squash to pull apart the flesh into spaghetti-like strands.
3. Transfer the spaghetti squash strands into a large mixing bowl.

Step 4: Combine and Assemble

1. Add the seasoned vegan cheese mixture to the spaghetti squash and toss well to ensure all the strands are evenly coated with the cheese and seasoning.
2. Transfer the cheesy spaghetti squash mixture to a baking dish.

Step 5: Bake the Spaghetti Squash

1. **Sprinkle the remaining vegan parmesan cheese** on top of the spaghetti squash mixture.
2. **Bake the dish** in the preheated oven for an additional 10-15 minutes, or until the cheese is melted and bubbly.
3. For an extra golden crust, you can place it under the broiler for 2-3 minutes but watch it closely to avoid burning.

Step 6: Garnish and Serve

1. Once baked, remove the dish from the oven and let it cool slightly.
2. Garnish with some fresh parsley and an extra sprinkle of vegan parmesan if desired.
3. Serve and enjoy this savory, cheesy vegan baked spaghetti squash dish!

HEALING AND NUTRITION

Spaghetti squash is a nutrient-rich, low-calorie alternative to traditional pasta, making this dish a perfect meal for those on a weight-loss journey. The natural **fiber** content in spaghetti squash aids digestion and promotes a feeling of fullness, helping to curb overeating.

By using **vegan cheese** and **vegan parmesan**, this recipe is entirely dairy-free, which reduces inflammation and helps many individuals avoid bloating and digestive discomfort that can come with consuming dairy. Choosing plant-based ingredients also lowers unhealthy fat intake, supporting heart health and weight management.

People who have switched to meals like this baked spaghetti squash have noticed improvements in their energy levels, weight loss, and overall well-being. The combination of low-carb spaghetti squash and **nutrient-packed herbs** such as oregano and parsley provides a flavorful and healthy alternative to traditional cheesy pasta dishes without sacrificing taste.

This dish is satisfying yet light, giving people the ability to enjoy their meals without guilt while supporting their journey to a healthier lifestyle.

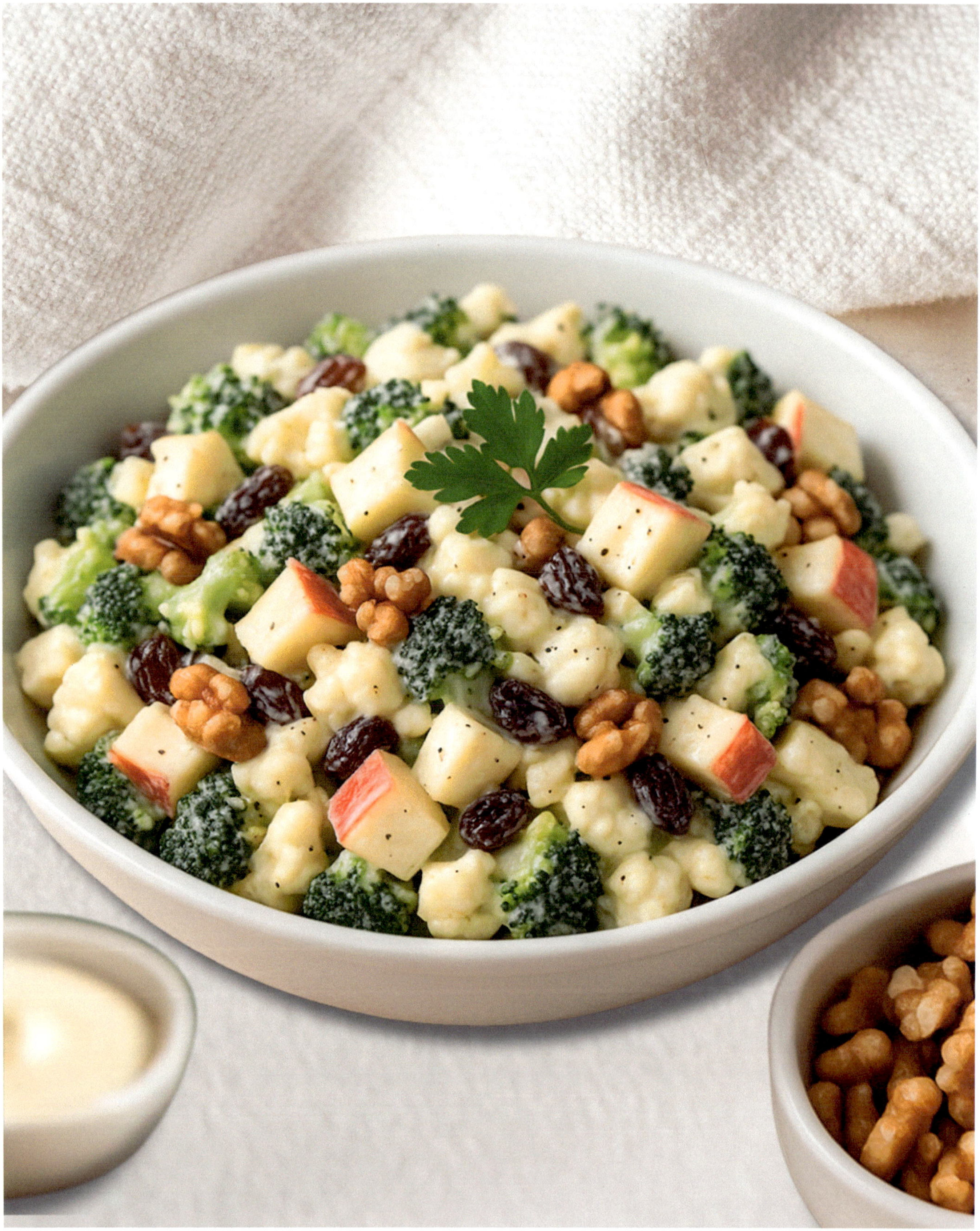

VEGAN WALDORF SALAD

WITH BROCCOLI, CAULIFLOWER, AND APPLES

INGREDIENTS:

- 1 cup broccoli florets (chopped into small pieces)
- 1 cup cauliflower florets (chopped into small pieces)
- 2 medium apples (cored and diced, use a crisp variety like Granny Smith or Honeycrisp)
- 1/2 cup walnuts (roughly chopped)
- 1/2 cup vegan mayonnaise
- 1/4 cup raisins
- 1 tablespoon lemon juice (to prevent apples from browning and add freshness)
- Optional garnish: fresh parsley or additional walnuts
- Salt and pepper to taste

INSTRUCTIONS:

Prepare the Vegetables and Fruit

1. **Chop the broccoli and cauliflower** into small bite-sized florets.
2. **Core and dice the apples** into small cubes. For added freshness and to prevent browning, toss the apples in 1 tablespoon of lemon juice and set aside.

Prepare the Salad Base

1. In a large mixing bowl, combine the chopped broccoli, cauliflower, diced apples, chopped walnuts, and raisins.
2. Stir gently to distribute all the ingredients evenly.

Add the Dressing

1. Add the vegan mayonnaise to the salad mixture. Stir well to coat all the ingredients evenly with the mayo.
2. Season the salad with a pinch of salt and freshly ground black pepper to taste.

Chill and Serve

1. Cover the bowl and place it in the refrigerator for at least 30 minutes to allow the flavors to meld together.

2. Before serving, give the salad a quick stir, and garnish with additional walnuts or fresh parsley, if desired.

Serve and Enjoy

1. Serve your vegan Waldorf salad as a refreshing side dish, or enjoy it as a light, nutritious meal on its own.

HEALING AND NUTRITION

This vegan Waldorf salad is not only delicious but also offers a host of health benefits, particularly for those focused on weight loss and overall well-being. **Broccoli** and **cauliflower** are cruciferous vegetables rich in fiber, vitamins, and antioxidants, which support digestion, detoxification, and weight management. These vegetables are low in calories but high in nutrients, making them perfect for those looking to stay full and satisfied without overeating.

Apples, high in fiber and vitamin C, add natural sweetness and crunch to the salad, while helping to regulate blood sugar levels and curb cravings. The **walnuts** provide heart-healthy omega-3 fats and protein, which are essential for maintaining energy levels and promoting satiety.

By using **vegan mayonnaise** instead of traditional mayo, this salad avoids excess saturated fats, which can contribute to inflammation and weight gain. Those who have incorporated plant-based alternatives into their diet often find that they experience less bloating and more stable energy levels, which can greatly support weight loss efforts.

Many people who have turned to nutrient-dense, whole-food-based salads like this one have reported improvements in digestion, skin health, and sustainable weight loss. The combination of healthy fats, fiber, and plant-based protein makes this vegan Waldorf salad an ideal choice for those on a journey to better health.

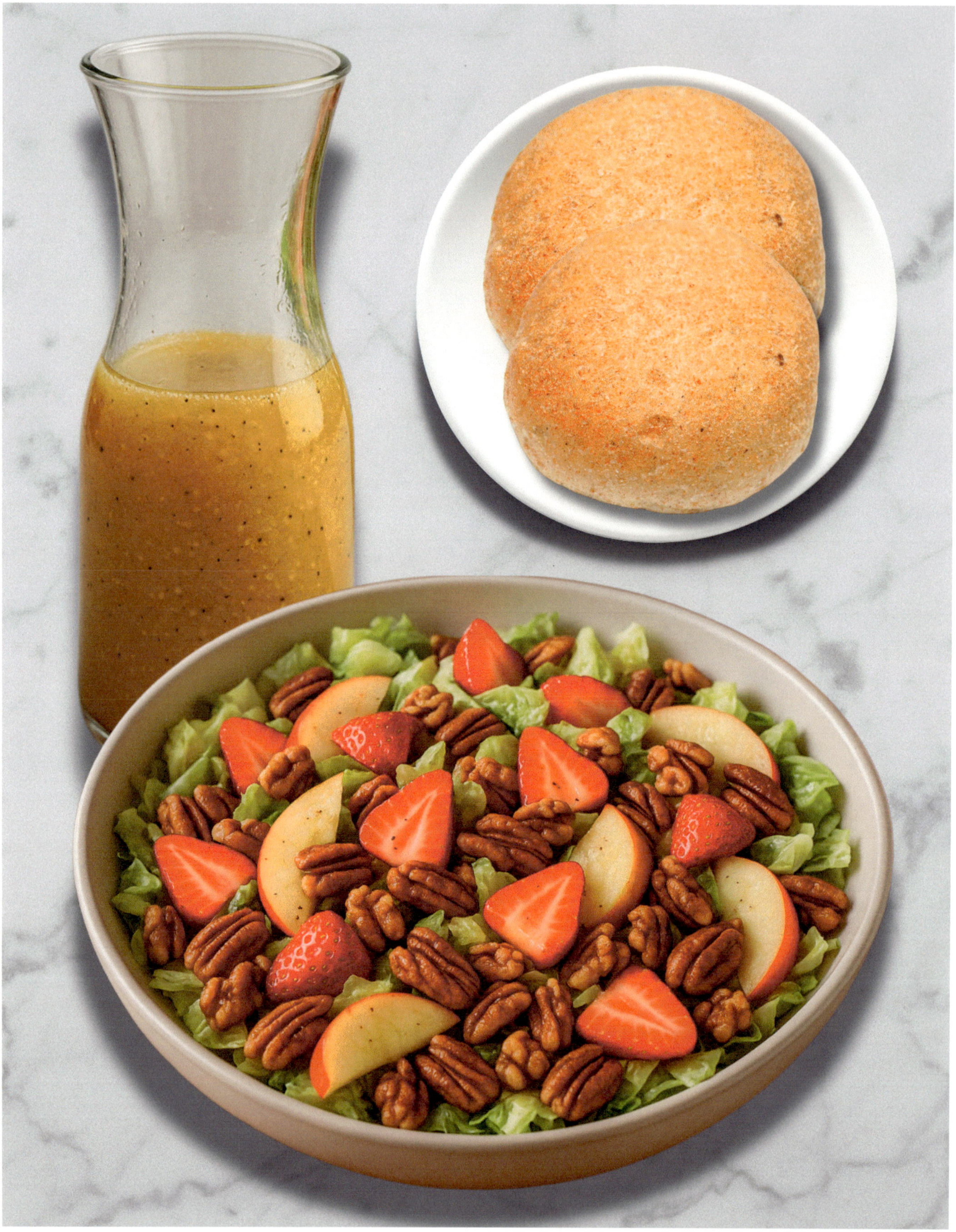

THE SADE: VEGAN STRAWBERRY WALNUT PECAN SALAD

INGREDIENTS:

- 1 head iceberg lettuce (chopped or torn into bite-sized pieces)
- 1/2 cup pecans (toasted)
- 1/2 cup walnuts (toasted)
- 1 medium apple (cored and thinly sliced)
- 2 tablespoons maple syrup
- 2 tablespoons lemon juice (freshly squeezed)
- 1 tablespoon apple cider vinegar
- 1 cup fresh strawberries (sliced)
- Salt and pepper to taste

INSTRUCTIONS:

Prepare the Salad Base

1. **Wash and chop the iceberg lettuce** into bite-sized pieces. Place the lettuce in a large salad bowl.
2. **Slice the strawberries** and **thinly slice the apples** (you can leave the peel on for extra fiber and nutrients). Add them to the lettuce.

Toast the Nuts

1. **Toast the pecans and walnuts** by placing them in a dry skillet over medium heat. Stir frequently for 3-5 minutes until they become golden and fragrant. Be careful not to burn them.
2. Let the toasted nuts cool slightly, then add them to the salad bowl.

Prepare the Dressing

1. In a small bowl or jar, whisk together the **maple syrup**, **lemon juice**, and **apple cider vinegar** until smooth and well combined.
2. Add a pinch of **salt and pepper** to taste.

Assemble the Salad

1. **Drizzle the dressing** over the salad, ensuring it coats all the ingredients evenly.
2. Toss gently to combine the lettuce, fruit, nuts, and dressing.

Serve

1. Serve immediately for the freshest flavor and crunch.
2. Optionally, garnish with extra toasted nuts or fresh herbs like mint for a more refreshing touch.

HEALING AND NUTRITION

This **Strawberry Walnut Pecan Salad** is a nutritious, delicious meal that supports healing and weight loss through its wholesome ingredients. **Strawberries** are high in antioxidants and vitamin C, helping the body fight free radicals, reduce inflammation, and boost immune function. Their natural sweetness also satisfies sugar cravings without the need for processed sugars, supporting weight management.

Walnuts and **pecans** are loaded with healthy fats, omega-3s, and protein, which promote satiety and reduce overeating. These nuts also have anti-inflammatory properties and help balance blood sugar levels, making them great for anyone looking to improve their metabolic health and lose weight.

Apples provide fiber and natural sweetness while being low in calories. Fiber aids digestion, and apples are known for promoting gut health, which is key to healthy weight loss.

The dressing, made with **maple syrup**, **lemon juice**, and **apple cider vinegar**, offers a balance of sweet, tangy flavors while avoiding unhealthy fats. **Apple cider vinegar** is well-known for its ability to support weight loss by improving metabolism and regulating blood sugar.

Many people who have made this salad a regular part of their diet have experienced improved digestion, more stable energy levels, and a satisfying meal that aids in weight loss. The combination of healthy fats, fiber, and fresh fruits provides both nourishment and flavor, making it an ideal addition to a weight-loss journey.

VEGAN
Side Dishes

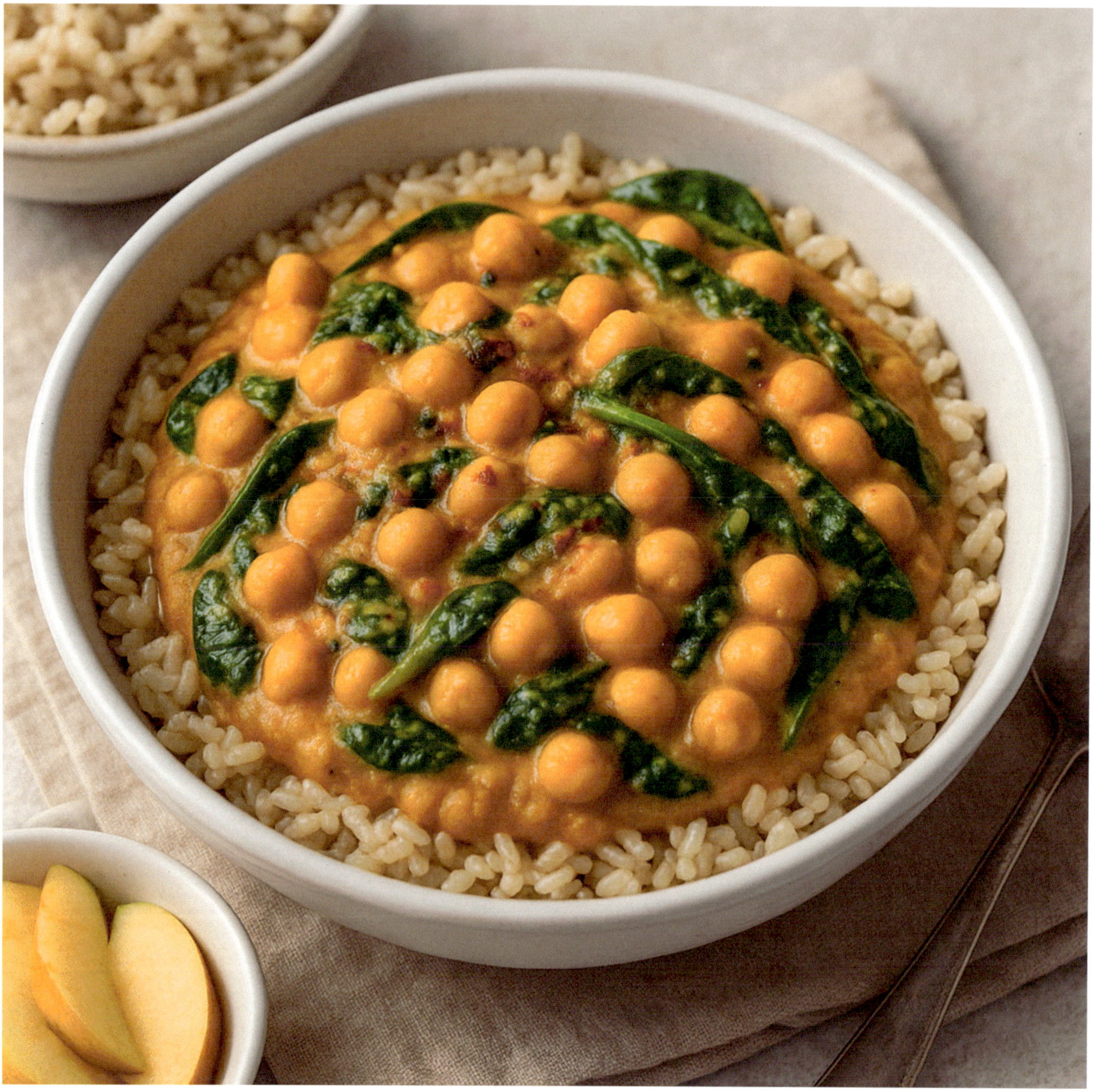

VEGAN CHICKPEA CURRY

This hearty vegan chickpea curry is packed with flavors from ginger, garlic, and warm spices like cinnamon and paprika. The creamy coconut milk base combined with nutrient-dense spinach and protein-rich chickpeas makes this dish both satisfying and nutritious. Perfect for a comforting meal that's good for both healing and weight management.

INGREDIENTS

- 1 medium onion, finely chopped
- 3 cloves garlic, grated or minced
- 1 tbsp fresh ginger, grated
- 2 tbsp olive oil
- 1 can (15 oz) chickpeas, drained and rinsed
- 1 can (14 oz) coconut milk
- 2 cups fresh spinach
- 1 tsp onion powder
- 1 tsp crushed red pepper (optional, for heat)
- 1 tsp paprika
- ¼ tsp ground cinnamon
- Salt and black pepper to taste

INSTRUCTIONS

Sauté the Aromatics

1. **Heat the Oil**: In a large skillet or pot, heat the olive oil over medium heat.
2. **Cook the Onions**: Add the chopped onions and cook for about 5 minutes until soft and translucent.
3. **Add Garlic and Ginger**: Stir in the grated garlic and ginger, and sauté for another 2 minutes until fragrant.

Add the Spices

1. **Spice It Up**: Add the crushed red pepper, onion powder, paprika, cinnamon, salt, and black pepper. Stir the spices into the onion mixture and cook for 1 minute to allow the spices to bloom and enhance the flavors.

Add Chickpeas and Coconut Milk

1. **Combine Chickpeas and Coconut Milk**: Add the chickpeas and coconut milk to the skillet. Stir well to combine all the ingredients. Let the mixture simmer for 10 minutes over medium-low heat, allowing the flavors to meld and the sauce to thicken slightly.

Add the Spinach

1. **Wilt the Spinach**: Stir in the fresh spinach leaves. Cook for another 3-5 minutes until the spinach wilts and becomes tender.

Adjust and Serve

1. **Taste and Adjust**: Taste the curry and adjust the seasoning as needed. Add more salt, pepper, or crushed red pepper for extra heat.
2. **Serve**: Serve the chickpea curry over brown rice, quinoa, or with flatbread for a complete meal.

HEALING AND NUTRITION

This vegan chickpea curry is not just a flavorful dish; it has also become a favorite for those focused on healing and weight loss. Chickpeas are a fantastic plant-based protein source that helps you feel full for longer, while spinach provides essential vitamins and minerals like iron and vitamin K. Coconut milk adds creaminess but is still lighter compared to many dairy-based sauces.

One person who adopted a plant-based diet found that by adding this chickpea curry to their meal rotation helped them manage their weight and feel more energized. By replacing heavier, meat-based curries with this plant-based version, they were able to cut down on excess calories while still enjoying the rich and comforting flavors they loved.

The combination of fiber from chickpeas and spinach, along with healthy fats from olive oil and coconut milk, helped them stay full longer, reducing the temptation to snack between meals. Over time, this led to a weight loss of 10 pounds in just two months. Additionally, the anti-inflammatory properties of ingredients like garlic, ginger, and cinnamon supported their overall healing process, reducing bloating and digestive discomfort.

By focusing on plant-based, whole foods like chickpeas, spinach, and coconut milk, they were able to nourish their body while enjoying a satisfying and flavorful meal. This recipe is perfect for anyone looking to embrace a healthier lifestyle while still enjoying delicious, comforting food.

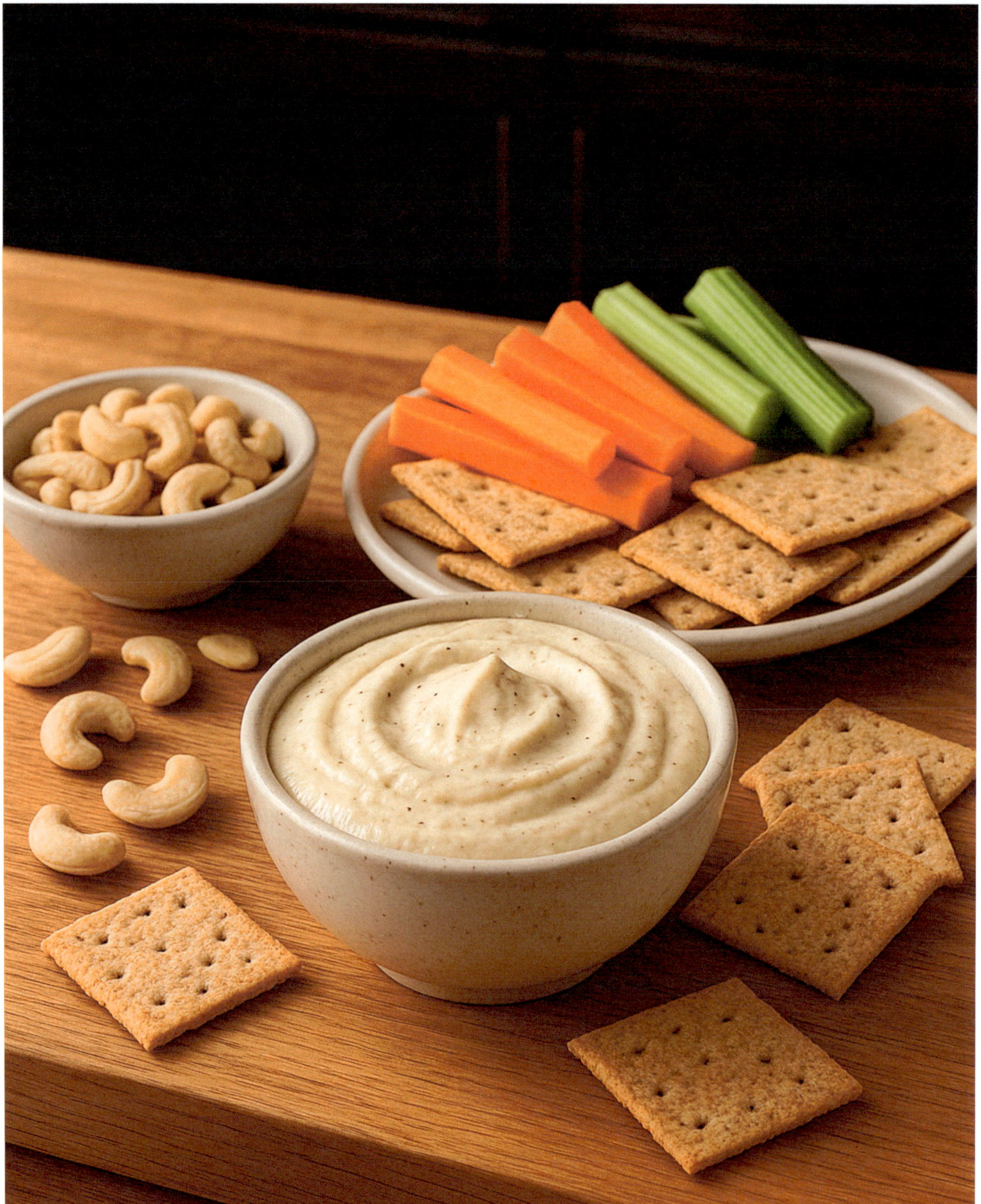

VEGAN CASHEW CHEESE (HALVED CASHEWS)

This simple vegan cashew cheese recipe is creamy, tangy, and versatile. Made with cashews, lemon, nutritional yeast, and garlic, it is perfect for spreading, dipping, or using in various dishes. It is a healthier alternative to traditional cheese, rich in plant-based fats and nutrients.

INGREDIENTS

- ½ cup cashews (soaked in water for at least 4 hours or overnight)
- 1 tbsp lemon juice (freshly squeezed)
- 1 garlic clove (or more if you like it garlicky)
- 1 tsp garlic powder
- ¼ cup water (adjust for desired consistency)
- 1 tsp garlic powder
- 2 tbsp nutritional yeast (for a cheesy flavor)
- ¼ tsp salt (adjust to taste)
- 2 tbsp olive oil

INSTRUCTIONS

Prepare the Cashews

1. **Soak the Cashews**: Soak the cashews in water for at least 4 hours or overnight to soften them. This will make them easier to blend and create a smoother texture.
2. **Drain the Cashews**: Once soaked, drain and rinse the cashews thoroughly.

Blend the Ingredients

1. **Add to Blender**: Place the soaked cashews, lemon juice, garlic clove, garlic powder, nutritional yeast, salt, olive oil, and water into a blender or food processor.
2. **Blend**: Blend on high until the mixture is smooth and creamy. You may need to stop and scrape down the sides a few times to ensure everything is evenly blended.
   - **Adjust Consistency**: If the mixture is too thick, add more water, a tablespoon at a time, until you reach your desired consistency. If you prefer a firmer cheese, use less water.

Taste and Adjust

1. **Taste**: Taste the cashew cheese and adjust seasoning as needed. Add more salt, lemon, or nutritional yeast depending on your flavor preferences.

2. **Optional**: For a firmer, more "aged" cheese texture, you can refrigerate the cashew cheese for 1-2 hours before serving.

Serve

1. **Serve**: Use this vegan cashew cheese as a spread for crackers, in sandwiches, or as a dip for veggies. It is also great as a topping for salads, pasta, or pizza!

HEALING AND NUTRITION

This vegan cashew cheese has become a favorite among those seeking healthier, plant-based alternatives to traditional dairy products. Cashews are rich in healthy fats, magnesium, and protein, making them an excellent choice for those looking to nourish their bodies while enjoying a creamy and cheesy flavor.

One person shared how transitioning to a plant-based diet, including making their own cashew cheese, helped them shed extra pounds and improve their overall health. By replacing high-calorie dairy cheeses with this nutrient-dense vegan alternative, they were able to reduce their intake of saturated fats and avoid the bloating and discomfort often associated with dairy.

The combination of cashews, garlic, and nutritional yeast in this recipe provides a satisfying flavor without relying on processed ingredients. Over the course of three months, this person lost 8 pounds while incorporating cashew cheese into their meals. They noticed improvements in their digestion, clearer skin, and more consistent energy levels.

Cashews are also a good source of heart-healthy monounsaturated fats, which can help reduce bad cholesterol levels. The lemon and garlic in the recipe not only add flavor but also offer anti-inflammatory and immune-boosting benefits, supporting overall health. This recipe is a perfect example of how making small, mindful substitutions can contribute to both healing and weight loss while still enjoying flavorful, comforting food!

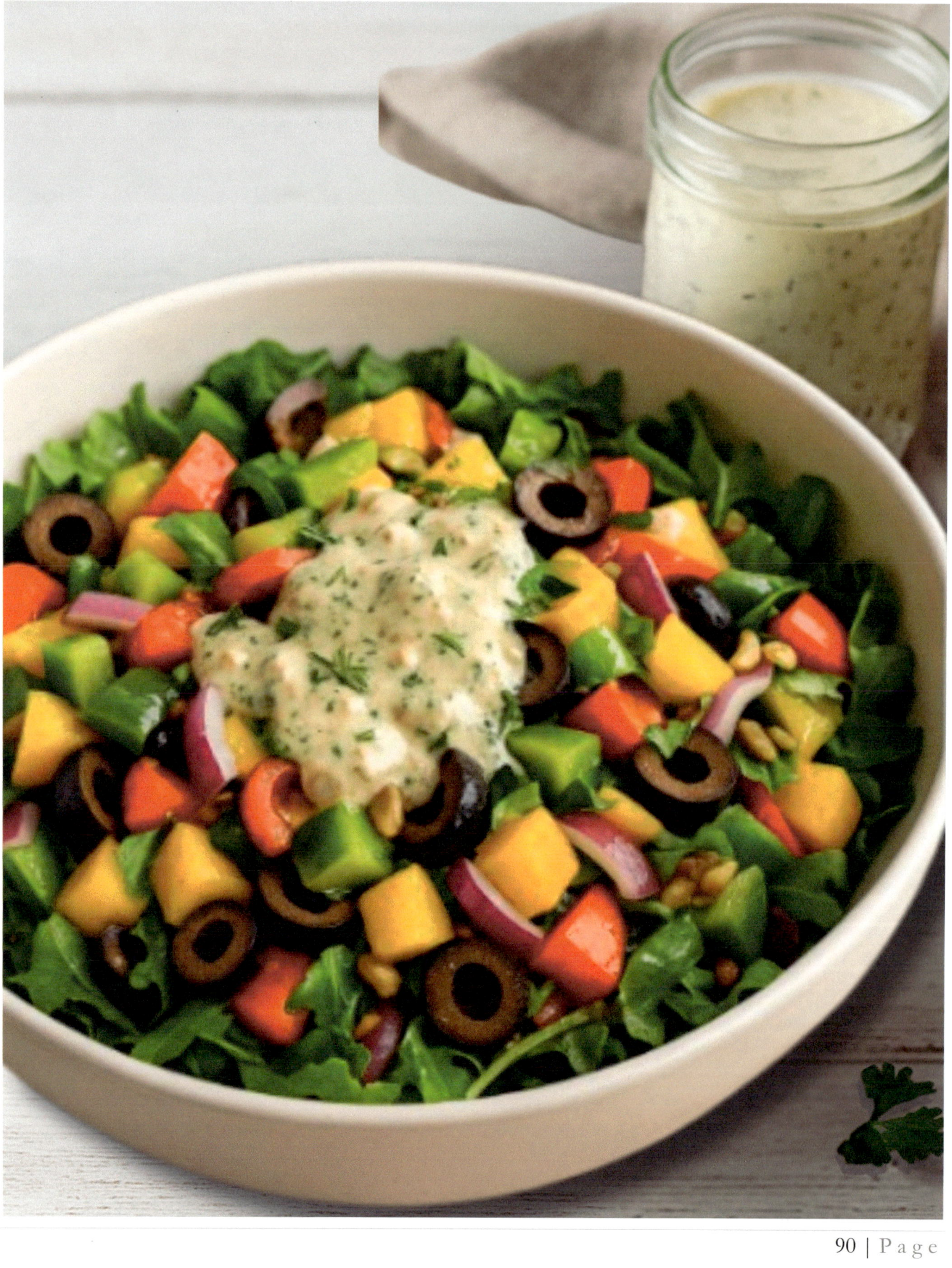

VEGAN VEGGIE SALAD

This vibrant and nutrient-packed vegan veggie salad is loaded with fresh greens, peppers, onions, and olives, offering a satisfying mix of textures and flavors. The cashew and dill dressing adds a creamy, tangy twist, making this salad a wholesome and filling meal.

INGREDIENTS

Salad Ingredients

- 2 cups arugula
- 1 cup red lettuce, chopped
- 1 cup green lettuce, chopped
- ½ red onion, thinly sliced
- 1 green bell pepper, chopped
- 1 yellow bell pepper, chopped
- 1 red bell pepper, chopped
- ½ cup black olives, sliced
- 1-2 tomatoes, chopped
- Salt and black pepper to taste
- 1-2 garlic cloves, minced

Dressing Ingredients

- ½ cup raw cashews, chopped
- 2 tbsp fresh dill, finely chopped
- 2 garlic cloves, minced
- ½ tsp onion powder
- ½ tsp paprika
- ¼ tsp black pepper
- 2-3 tbsp water (to adjust consistency)
- Salt to taste

INSTRUCTIONS

Prepare the Salad

- **Wash the Greens**: Rinse the arugula, red lettuce, and green lettuce under cold water. Pat dry or spin them in a salad spinner to remove excess moisture.
- **Chop the Vegetables**: Slice the red onions, chop the bell peppers (green, yellow, and red), and tomatoes. Slice the black olives.
- **Combine in a Bowl**: Place the arugula, red lettuce, and green lettuce into a large salad bowl. Add the chopped veggies (onions, peppers, tomatoes, olives) on top.
- **Season**: Sprinkle the salad with a pinch of salt, freshly ground black pepper, and minced garlic.

Prepare the Dressing

- **Chop the Cashews**: Finely chop the raw cashews or pulse them briefly in a food processor.
- **Mix the Dressing**: In a small bowl, combine the chopped cashews, fresh dill, minced garlic, onion powder, paprika, and black pepper. Gradually add water to reach a creamy consistency, stirring as you go. Add salt to taste and adjust the water to your desired thickness.

Toss the Salad

- **Drizzle the Dressing:** Pour the creamy cashew and dill dressing over the veggie salad.
- **Toss:** Gently toss the salad to ensure all the vegetables are evenly coated with the dressing.
- **Serve:** Serve immediately or chill the salad for 10-15 minutes to let the flavors meld together.

HEALING AND NUTRITION

This vegan veggie salad is an incredible blend of nutrient-dense ingredients that support both healing and weight loss. Arugula and lettuce provide a low-calorie base while being rich in fiber and antioxidants, helping to boost digestion and reduce inflammation. The peppers, onions, and tomatoes are high in vitamins A, C, and E, which support the immune system and promote skin health.

One person who regularly added this salad to their diet shared how it helped them lose weight and improve their overall well-being. By switching to a plant-based, whole-food diet and including this veggie salad in their meals, they experienced better digestion and sustained energy levels throughout the day. The high fiber content from vegetables and greens helped them feel full longer, reducing overeating and cravings for unhealthy snacks.

In two months of including this salad as part of their lunch routine, they lost 10 pounds. Healthy fats from the cashew-based dressing provided satiety without the heaviness of traditional, oil-laden dressings, helping them cut down on unnecessary calories. Additionally, the fresh dill and garlic offered detoxifying and anti-inflammatory benefits, which contributed to improved gut health and overall vitality.

This nutrient-packed salad offers a satisfying, delicious, and clean way to fuel the body while supporting weight loss and promoting healing from the inside out.

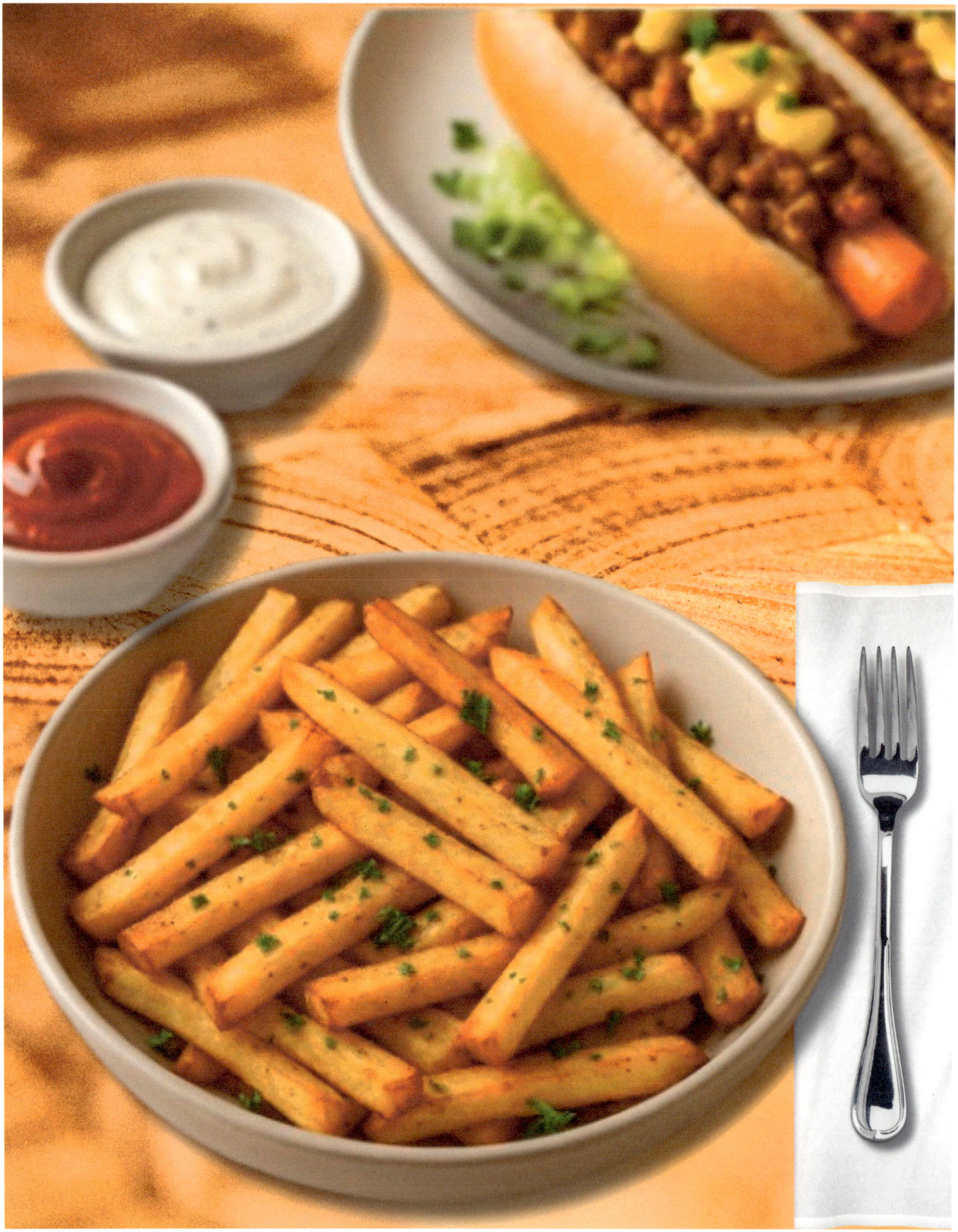

VEGAN FRENCH FRIES

These vegan french fries are a healthier take on the classic snack, made with grapeseed oil, a neutral, heart-healthy option. With a touch of garlic powder, salt, and black pepper, they are flavorful, crispy, and perfect for a quick, satisfying treat.

INGREDIENTS:

- 4 medium potatoes (russet or Yukon gold work best)
- 3 tablespoons grapeseed oil
- 1 teaspoon garlic powder
- Optional: fresh herbs like parsley or rosemary for garnish
- 1/2 teaspoon black pepper
- 1/2 teaspoon salt (or to taste)

INSTRUCTIONS:

Prepare the Potatoes:

- Wash and peel the potatoes (you can leave the skin on if you prefer extra fiber).
- Cut the potatoes into thin strips, about 1/4-inch thick for crispy fries, or thicker for a more classic french fry texture.

Soak the Potatoes:

- Place the sliced potatoes into a bowl of cold water and let them soak for at least 30 minutes. This removes excess starch and helps the fries become crispier when cooked.
- After soaking, drain and pat the potatoes dry with a kitchen towel or paper towel.

Preheat the Oven (or Air Fryer):

- Preheat the oven to 425°F (220°C) if baking. If using an air fryer, preheat it to 375°F (190°C).

Season the Fries:

- In a large bowl, toss the dried potato slices with the grapeseed oil, garlic powder, salt, and black pepper. Make sure each fry is evenly coated.

Bake or Air-Fry the Fries:

- **Oven Method**: Spread the fries in a single layer on a baking sheet lined with parchment paper or foil. Bake for 30-40 minutes, flipping halfway through, until golden brown and crispy. For extra crispiness, broil for the last 2-3 minutes.
- **Air Fryer Method**: Arrange the fries in the air fryer basket in a single layer. Fry for 20-25 minutes, shaking the basket halfway through, until golden and crispy.

Serve:

- Once the fries are done, sprinkle a little more salt and pepper if desired. Optionally, garnish with freshly chopped herbs like parsley or rosemary for extra flavor.

Enjoy:

- Serve immediately with your favorite vegan dipping sauces like ketchup, vegan mayo, or mustard.

HEALING AND NUTRITION

TESTIMONIAL: "*As someone who loves french fries but was looking for a healthier version, this recipe became a lifesaver! The use of grapeseed oil, which is rich in healthy fats and antioxidants, made me feel less guilty about indulging in my favorite comfort food. I noticed a huge difference in digestion and energy levels after switching to this healthier oil. By replacing deep-fried fries with this baked version, I have also managed to keep my weight in check without sacrificing taste. The garlic powder and black pepper add great flavor, and now these fries have become my go-to snack when I am craving something crispy but still health-conscious.*"

Health Benefits:

- **Grapeseed Oil**: A heart-healthy oil rich in polyunsaturated fats and vitamin E, which supports skin health and metabolism.
- **Potatoes**: A good source of fiber (when the skin is left on), potassium, and vitamins C and B6. They are filling without being high in calories, making them a great option for weight management.
- **Garlic Powder**: Provides a flavorful, anti-inflammatory boost that can also support heart health and metabolism.
- **Black Pepper**: Contains piperine, which may improve digestion and nutrient absorption, contributing to overall health.

This simple yet flavorful french fry recipe offers a healthier way to enjoy a classic comfort food while supporting weight loss and healing with wholesome ingredients.

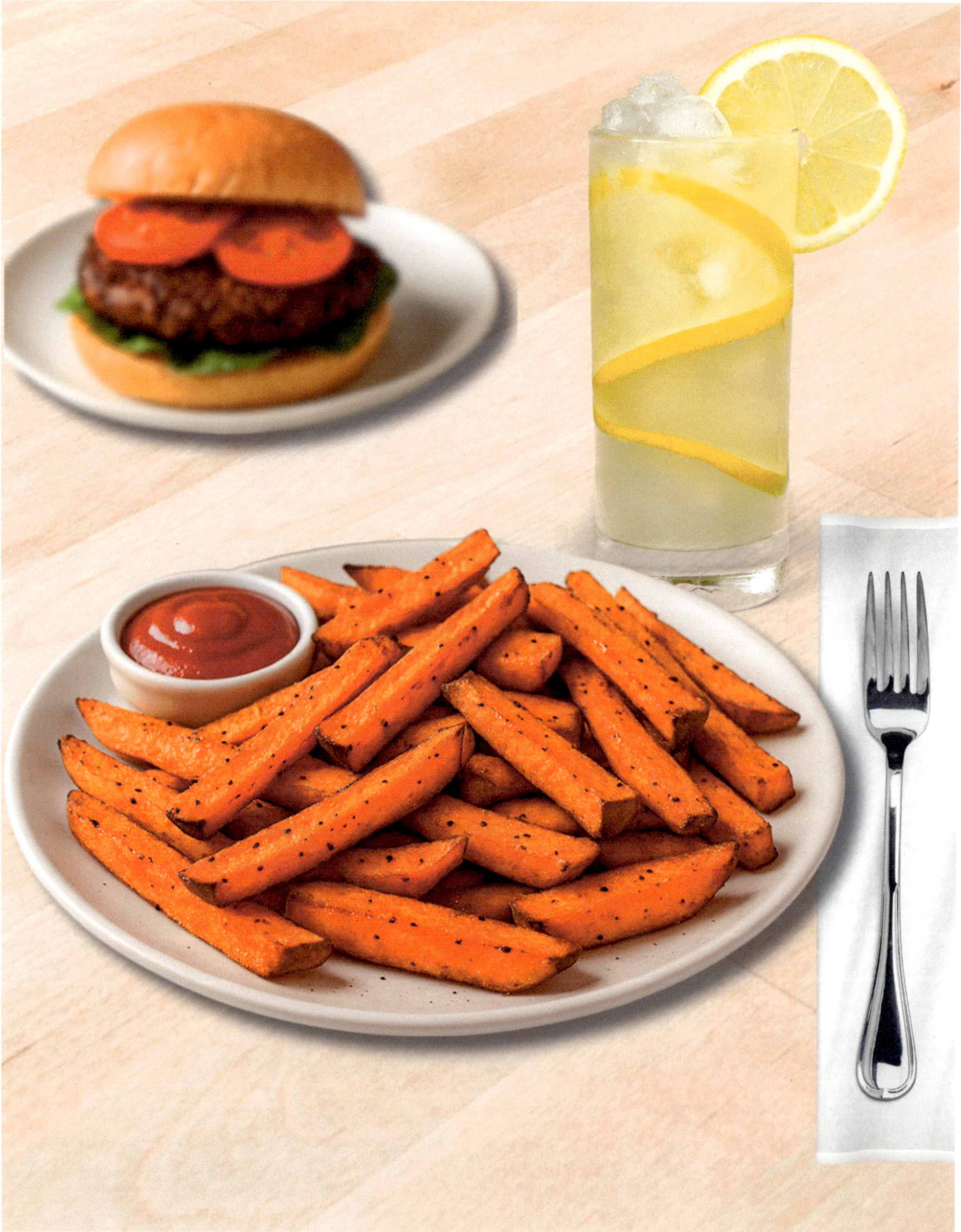

VEGAN SWEET POTATO FRIES

These delicious and crispy vegan sweet potato fries are packed with flavor and nutrients, making them a perfect guilt-free snack. Made with grapeseed oil, garlic powder, salt, and pepper, they are a healthier twist on regular fries, offering plenty of vitamins and minerals.

INGREDIENTS:

- 3 medium sweet potatoes
- 2-3 tablespoons grapeseed oil
- 1 teaspoon garlic powder
- 1/2 teaspoon salt (or to taste)
- 1/2 teaspoon black pepper
- Optional: paprika or cayenne for extra spice

INSTRUCTIONS:

Preheat the Oven (or Air Fryer):

- Preheat your oven to 425°F (220°C) if baking. If using an air fryer, preheat to 375°F (190°C).

Prepare the Sweet Potatoes:

- Wash and peel the sweet potatoes (optionally, you can leave the skin on for extra fiber).
- Slice the sweet potatoes into fries, about 1/4-inch thick. Try to keep the size consistent for even cooking.

Soak the Sweet Potatoes:

- Place the sliced sweet potatoes in a bowl of cold water and soak for at least 30 minutes. This helps remove excess starch, which leads to crispier fries.
- Drain and thoroughly pat the sweet potato slices dry with a kitchen towel or paper towels.

Season the Sweet Potatoes:

- In a large bowl, toss the dried sweet potato slices with grapeseed oil, garlic powder, salt, and black pepper. Make sure all the fries are evenly coated.
- For an extra kick, you can add a pinch of paprika or cayenne pepper at this step.

Bake or Air-Fry the Fries:

- **Oven Method**: Spread the sweet potato fries in a single layer on a baking sheet lined with parchment paper. Bake for 25-30 minutes, flipping halfway through. Bake until the fries are golden brown and crispy on the edges.
- **Air Fryer Method**: Place the fries in the air fryer basket in a single layer. Cook for 15-20 minutes, shaking halfway through, until crispy and cooked through.

Serve:

- Once the fries are golden and crispy, sprinkle a little more salt or pepper to taste. Serve immediately with your favorite vegan dips, such as avocado mayo, ketchup, or tahini sauce.

HEALING AND NUTRITION

TESTIMONIAL: "*I love sweet potatoes but always struggled to find a healthy way to satisfy my cravings for fries. This recipe was the perfect solution! The grapeseed oil kept them light and healthy while still giving me that crispy texture I love. The garlic powder added a great savory kick, and I felt full and satisfied without the heaviness that comes from traditional fries. Eating these sweet potato fries regularly as part of my meals made a huge difference in my digestion and energy levels. The high fiber content kept me full for longer, which helped me manage my weight and cut down on unnecessary snacking. Plus, they are packed with vitamins, so I felt like I was nourishing my body while enjoying something delicious.*"

Health Benefits:

- **Sweet Potatoes**: High in fiber, beta-carotene (vitamin A), vitamin C, and potassium. They help keep you full longer, promote healthy digestion, and can support weight management.
- **Grapeseed Oil**: A light oil rich in polyunsaturated fats and vitamin E, which supports heart health and skin health while helping to manage cholesterol levels.
- **Garlic Powder**: Adds flavor while also providing anti-inflammatory benefits and supporting the immune system.
- **Black Pepper**: Contains piperine, which helps improve nutrient absorption and supports digestion.

This vegan sweet potato fries recipe offers a nutritious and satisfying snack or side dish that aids in weight loss and promotes overall wellness without compromising on taste!

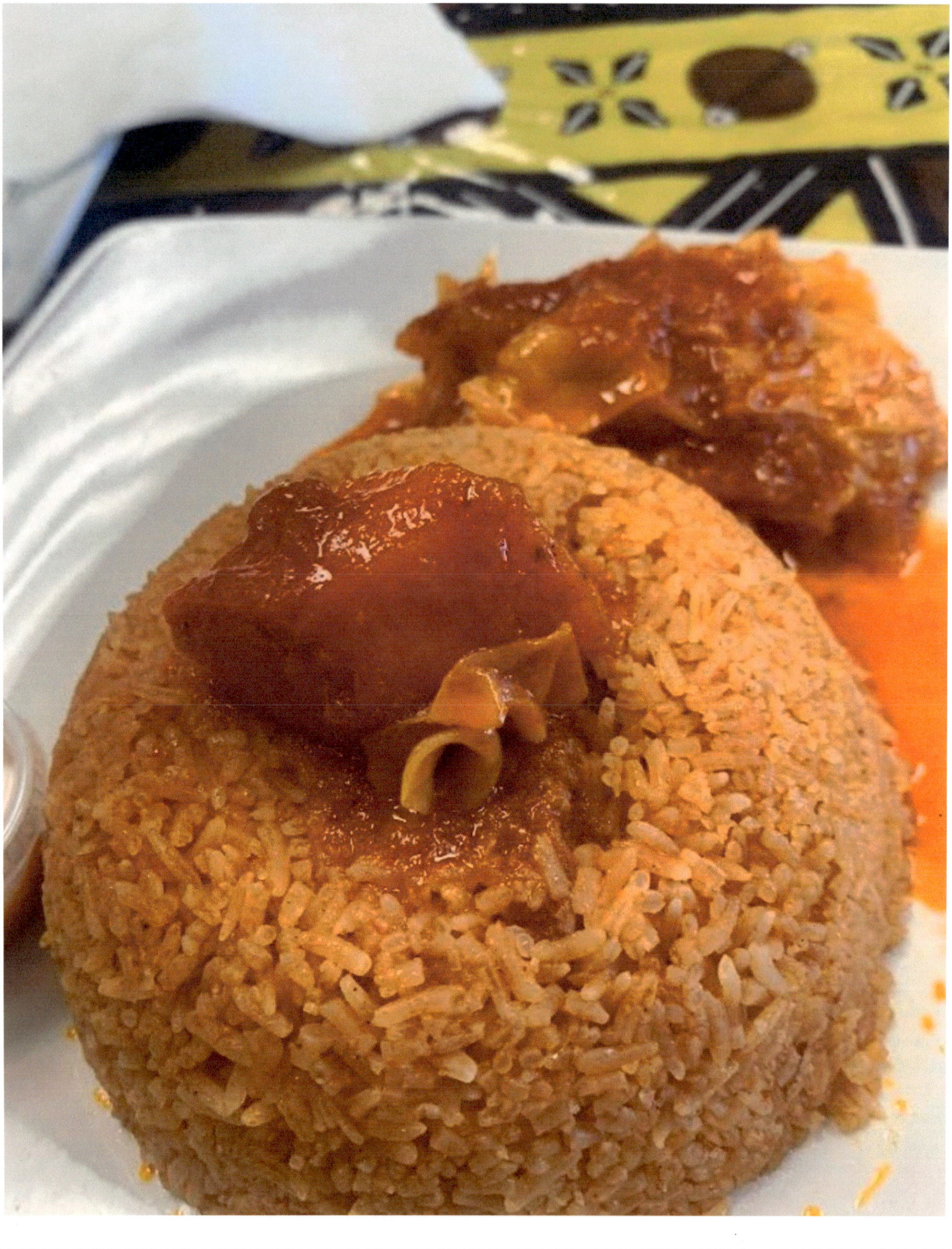

VEGAN JOLLOF RICE WITH CARROTS AND CABBAGE

This vibrant, flavorful vegan Jollof rice recipe is inspired by the classic West African dish, packed with spices, vegetables, and bold flavors. It is made with carrots, cabbage, and a rich tomato base, creating a hearty and satisfying meal. Palm oil adds richness, while scotch bonnet pepper gives it that traditional heat.

INGREDIENTS:

- 2 cups white rice (preferably long-grain)
- 1/4 cup of palm oil
- 1 large onion, diced
- 1 red bell pepper, diced
- 1-2 scotch bonnet peppers, minced (adjust for heat tolerance)
- 3 medium carrots, diced
- 1 small cabbage head, chopped
- 1/4 cup tomato paste
- 3 medium tomatoes, blended into a purée
- 2 bay leaves
- 4 cups of vegetable broth or water
- Salt and pepper to taste

INSTRUCTIONS:

Prepare the Ingredients:

- Wash the rice thoroughly under cold water until the water runs clear. This helps remove excess starch and prevents the rice from being too sticky.
- Blend the fresh tomatoes into a purée and set aside.

Sauté the Vegetables:

- Heat the palm oil in a large pot over medium heat. Once hot, add the diced onions and sauté until they become soft and translucent, about 4-5 minutes.
- Add the diced red pepper and minced scotch bonnet peppers. Stir and cook for another 2-3 minutes, allowing the flavors to blend and the peppers to soften.

Cook the Tomato Base:

- Stir in the tomato paste and cook for about 5 minutes, stirring occasionally, to reduce the acidity and bring out the sweetness of the tomato paste.
- Add the blended tomatoes and cook for another 10-15 minutes, stirring occasionally until the sauce reduces and thickens.

Add Carrots and Cabbage:

- Stir in the diced carrots and chopped cabbage. Cook for 5 minutes, allowing the vegetables to soften slightly.

Add Rice and Broth:

- Add the washed rice to the pot, stirring to combine it with the tomato and vegetable mixture. Make sure the rice is evenly coated.
- Add the vegetable broth (or water) and the bay leaves. Stir, then cover the pot and reduce the heat to low.
- Allow the rice to simmer for 25-30 minutes, stirring occasionally to prevent sticking. If the rice begins to dry before it is fully cooked, you can add a little more water or broth.

Check for Doneness:

- Once the rice is cooked and fluffy, remove the pot from the heat. Remove the bay leaves and fluff the rice with a fork.

Serve:

- Serve your vegan Jollof rice with additional vegetables or a side of plantains for a balanced meal. Enjoy hot!

HEALING AND NUTRITION

TESTIMONIAL: "*Jollof rice has always been one of my favorite dishes, but I wanted to make a version that would help support my wellness goals. This vegan recipe, loaded with carrots and cabbage, is not only delicious but also packed with nutrients. The carrots and cabbage were included to add texture, fiber, and vitamins, while the palm oil provides healthy fats that left me feeling satisfied. After incorporating this dish into my meal prep routine, I noticed a big improvement in my digestion and energy levels. The fiber-rich vegetables kept me full longer, helping me avoid unnecessary snacking. This hearty yet light meal has been perfect for my weight loss journey, while still letting me enjoy the bold flavors I love.*"

Health Benefits:

- **Carrots**: Rich in beta-carotene, fiber, and antioxidants, carrots support eye health, digestion, and weight loss by keeping you full longer.

- **Cabbage**: Low in calories but high in fiber, cabbage promotes gut health and weight management while providing essential vitamins like C and K.
- **White Rice**: A good source of energy, especially when paired with fiber-rich vegetables. Long-grain rice is less starchy and tends to keep its structure well.
- **Palm Oil**: A traditional ingredient in West African cooking, palm oil is rich in vitamin E and carotenoids, which are powerful antioxidants.
- **Scotch Bonnet Peppers**: High in capsaicin, these spicy peppers can boost metabolism and aid in fat burning, while adding depth of flavor to the dish.
- **Tomatoes and Tomato Paste**: Full of lycopene, an antioxidant that supports heart health and reduces inflammation.

This vegan Jollof rice recipe not only delivers on taste and tradition but also supports a healthy lifestyle with ingredients that aid in digestion, weight loss, and overall well-being.

VEGAN
Desserts

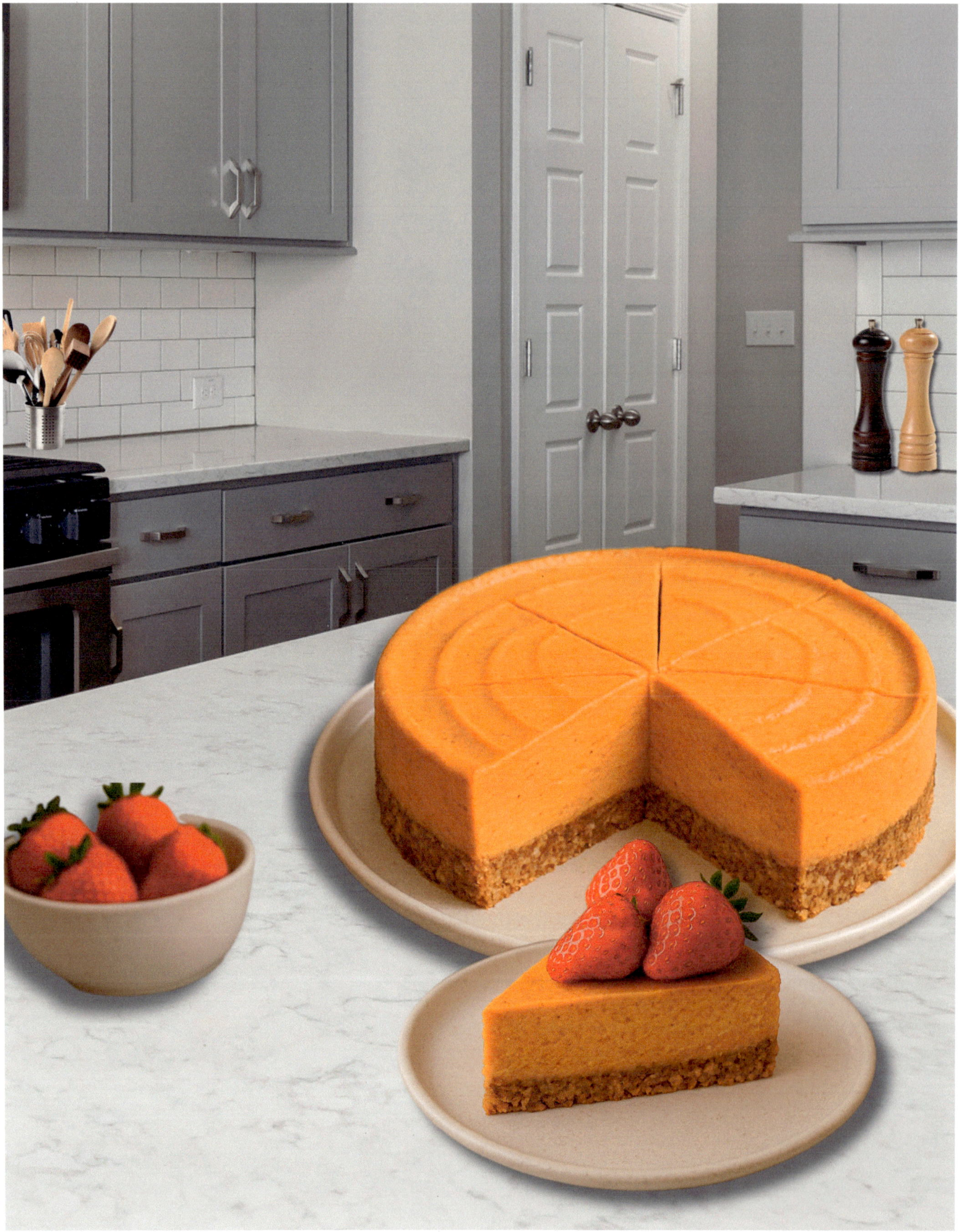

VEGAN SWEET POTATO CHEESECAKE (WITH VEGAN CRUST)

This vegan sweet potato cheesecake is creamy, rich, and made from wholesome ingredients like sweet potatoes, cashews, and coconut cream. It is completely plant-based and naturally sweetened, making it a healthier yet indulgent dessert. Perfect for anyone looking for a guilt-free treat that fits into their healing or weight-loss journey.

INGREDIENTS

For the Vegan Crust:

- 1 ½ cups of almond flour or finely ground oats
- ¼ cup melted organic vegan butter (or melted coconut oil)
- 1 tsp vanilla extract
- Pinch of sea salt
- 2 tbsp agave syrup or maple syrup

For the Cheesecake Filling:

- 2 medium sweet potatoes, baked or steamed and mashed
- 1 cup raw cashews (soaked for at least 2 hours or overnight, then drained)
- 1 can (14 oz) coconut cream
- ½ cup almond milk (unsweetened)
- ½ cup agave syrup (or maple syrup)
- 1 tsp cinnamon
- 2 tsp vanilla extract
- ¼ tsp nutmeg
- 2 tbsp lemon juice
- Pinch of sea salt

INSTRUCTIONS

Prepare the Vegan Crust

1. **Mix the Crust Ingredients**: In a bowl, combine almond flour (or ground oats) with melted vegan butter (or coconut oil), agave syrup, vanilla extract, and a pinch of sea salt. Stir until the mixture becomes a moist, crumbly texture.
2. **Form the Crust**: Press the mixture into the bottom of an 8-inch springform pan. Use the back of a spoon or your fingers to press it down evenly and firmly to create a compact layer. Place the crust in the freezer to set while you prepare the cheesecake filling.

Make the Cheesecake Filling

1. **Blend the Cashews and Sweet Potatoes**: In a high-speed blender or food processor, blend the soaked cashews, mashed sweet potatoes, and coconut cream until smooth.
2. **Add Flavorings**: Add almond milk, agave syrup, vanilla extract, cinnamon, nutmeg, lemon juice, and a pinch of sea salt to the blender. Continue blending until the mixture is silky smooth. Taste and adjust the sweetness or spices, if needed.

Assemble the Cheesecake

1. **Pour the Filling**: Pour the sweet potato cheesecake filling over the prepared crust. Smooth out the top with a spatula to create an even layer.
2. **Chill to Set**: Place the cheesecake in the refrigerator for at least 4-6 hours, or overnight, to allow the cheesecake to firm up.

Serve

Once set, carefully remove the cheesecake from the spring-form pan. Slice and serve as is, or garnish with a sprinkle of cinnamon, a drizzle of agave syrup, or coconut whipped cream.

HEALING AND NUTRITION

This vegan sweet potato cheesecake has become a beloved recipe for many who are on a healing and weight-loss journey. By removing processed sugars, refined oils, and dairy, this dessert offers a nutrient-dense alternative to traditional cheesecakes.

One individual shared how this recipe helped them transition to a plant-based diet, supporting their weight loss efforts. After years of struggling with cravings for sugary desserts, they discovered that the natural sweetness of sweet potatoes and agave satisfied their sweet tooth while offering valuable nutrients like fiber and vitamins A and C. Sweet potatoes are also known for their low glycemic index, helping to regulate blood sugar levels and prevent energy crashes.

Cashews, with their healthy fats and protein, provided satiety, reducing the need for frequent snacking. The inclusion of heart-healthy coconut cream and almond milk added a luscious, creamy texture without the cholesterol found in traditional dairy-based cheesecakes.

By incorporating this vegan cheesecake into their diet, they were able to enjoy a dessert that felt indulgent without hindering their health goals. Over several months, they noticed improvements in digestion, reduced inflammation, and a weight loss of over 15 pounds. The natural ingredients in this cheesecake, combined with a balanced plant-based diet, offered the nourishment their body needed for healing and weight management.

This cheesecake recipe is a testament to how delicious, nutrient-rich food can be a powerful tool for healing and achieving long-term health!

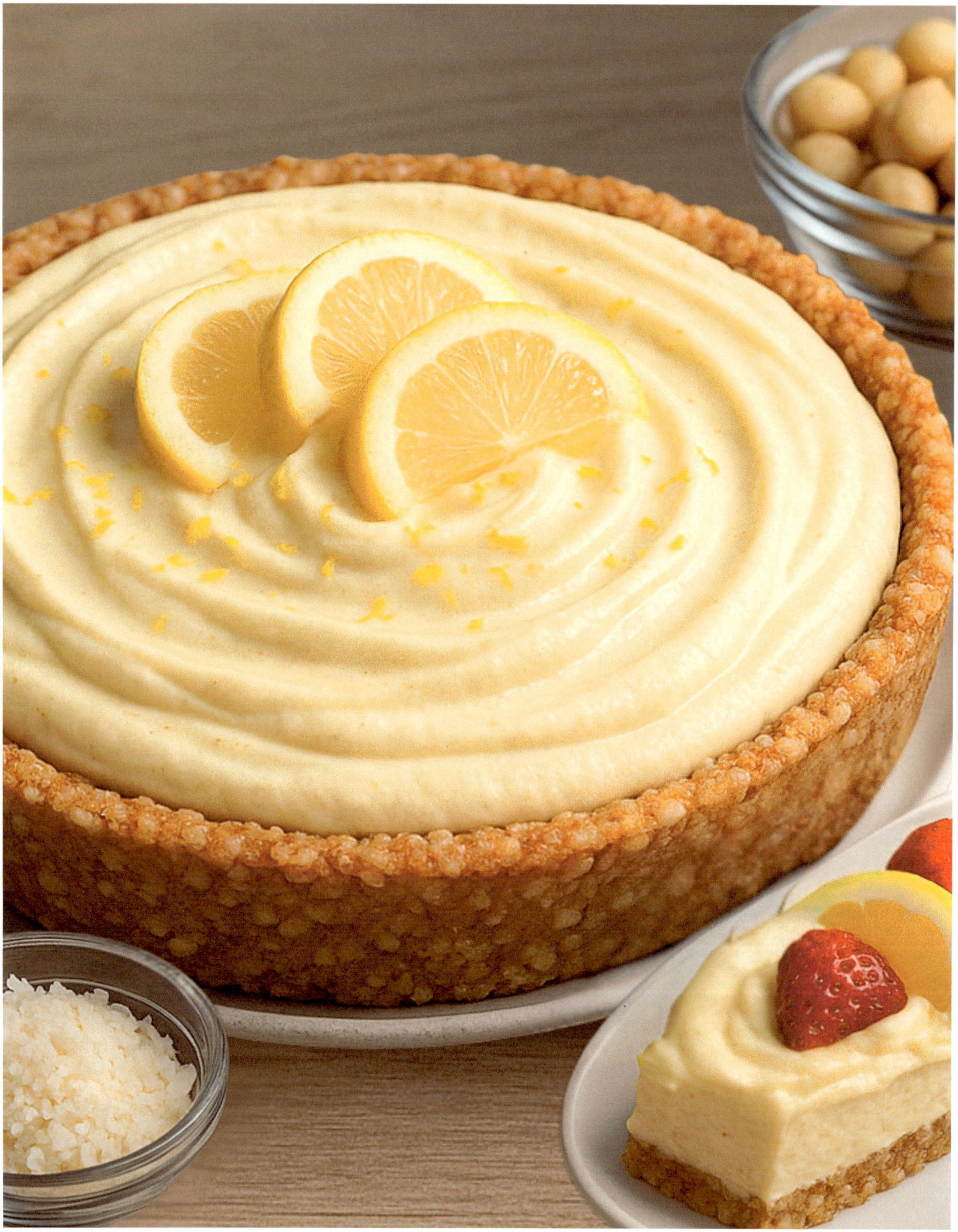

VEGAN LEMON WHIPPED MOUSSE

This light and refreshing vegan lemon whipped mousse is a perfect balance of creamy and tangy, made with nourishing, plant-based ingredients like coconut cream, agave, and fresh lemons. Paired with a crunchy macadamia nut and oat pie crust, it is both a decadent dessert and a healthy, healing treat.

INGREDIENTS

For the Macadamia Nut and Oat Pie Crust:

- 1 cup macadamia nuts
- ¾ cup oats (gluten-free if needed)
- ½ cup shredded unsweetened coconut
- 3 tbsp agave syrup
- 2 tbsp coconut oil (melted)
- Pinch of sea salt

- **For the Lemon Whipped Mousse:**

- 1 can (14 oz) coconut cream (chilled in the fridge overnight)
- ¼ cup agave syrup (or to taste)
- Zest and juice of 2 large lemons
- 1 tsp vanilla extract
- Pinch of sea salt

INSTRUCTIONS

Prepare the Pie Crust

1. **Process the Dry Ingredients**: In a food processor, combine the macadamia nuts, oats, and shredded coconut. Pulse until the mixture forms a coarse crumb texture, but do not over-process. You want a bit of crunch.
2. **Add Wet Ingredients**: Add the agave syrup, melted coconut oil, and a pinch of sea salt to the processor. Pulse until the mixture holds together when pressed between your fingers.
3. **Form the Crust**: Press the mixture evenly into the bottom and slightly up the sides of an 8-inch tart or pie pan. Use your fingers or the back of a spoon to create a compact, even layer.
4. **Chill the Crust**: Place the crust in the freezer while you prepare the lemon mousse filling.

Make the Lemon Whipped Mousse

1. **Prepare the Coconut Cream**: Open the chilled can of coconut cream and scoop out the thick, solid cream that has risen to the top (discard the liquid or save it for another recipe like smoothies).

2. **Whip the Coconut Cream**: In a large mixing bowl, use an electric hand mixer or stand mixer to whip the coconut cream on medium-high speed until light and fluffy, about 3-5 minutes.
3. **Add Lemon and Sweetener**: Add the agave syrup, lemon zest, lemon juice, vanilla extract, and a pinch of sea salt to the whipped coconut cream. Continue whipping for another minute until combined and fluffy.
4. **Taste and Adjust**: Taste the mousse and adjust the sweetness or lemon flavor by adding more agave or lemon juice, depending on your preference.

Assemble the Dessert

1. **Fill the Crust**: Spoon the whipped lemon mousse into the prepared pie crust, spreading it out evenly with a spatula.
2. **Chill**: Place the assembled mousse pie in the refrigerator for at least 2 hours (or longer) to allow the mousse to firm up and for the flavors to meld together.

Serve

Once set, slice and serve your vegan lemon whipped mousse pie. Garnish with extra lemon zest or shredded coconut for an added touch.

HEALING AND NUTRITION

This vegan lemon whipped mousse is more than just a delicious dessert; it is also a great choice for those on a healing journey or looking to manage their weight. The natural ingredients in this recipe, like coconut cream, lemon, and agave, are all nutrient-dense and free from processed sugars or dairy, making it much gentler on the digestive system.

One person who enjoyed this dessert as part of a plant-based diet found that it helped them reduce cravings for refined sugars and processed foods. The healthy fats from coconut cream and macadamia nuts provided satiety and energy, which helped them avoid overeating or snacking on less healthy options. Over time, they noticed improvements in their skin, digestion, and weight management. By cutting out heavy, dairy-based desserts and replacing them with lighter, plant-based alternatives, they were able to lose 10 pounds in two months while feeling energized and satisfied.

Lemons are also rich in vitamin C, which supports the immune system and helps with detoxification, while macadamia nuts and oats provide a blend of fiber, healthy fats, and plant-based proteins. Altogether, this mousse pie is not just a treat but a part of a balanced and nourishing diet that promotes healing and weight loss in a sustainable way.

The light and tangy flavors of this lemon mousse make it a refreshing option, perfect for when you want a dessert that leaves you feeling satisfied but not weighed down!

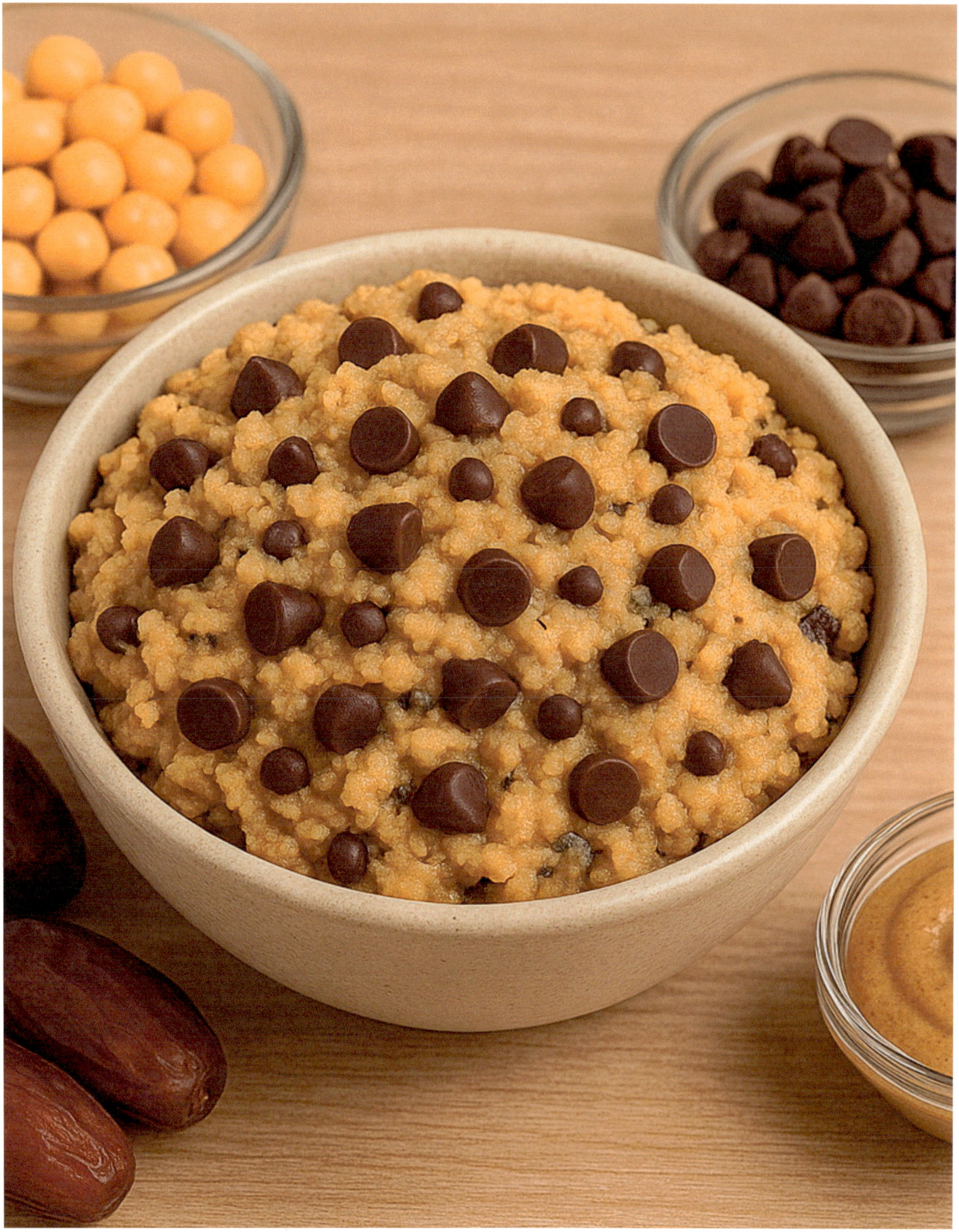

VEGAN CHICKPEA COOKIE DOUGH

This vegan chickpea cookie dough is a guilt-free treat made with wholesome ingredients like oat flour, chocolate chips, and naturally sweetened with dates. It is rich, satisfying, and completely safe to eat raw since it is made without eggs or dairy. Perfect for a healthy snack or dessert!

INGREDIENTS:

- 1 can (15 oz) chickpeas, drained and rinsed
- ½ cup oat flour (or blend rolled oats into flour)
- 6-8 pitted Medjool dates (soaked in warm water for 10 minutes if they are dry)
- 1 tsp vanilla extract
- ¼ cup dark chocolate chips (dairy-free)
- 2 tbsp almond butter or any nut/seed butter
- 1-2 tbsp almond milk (optional, to help with blending)

INSTRUCTIONS:

Prepare the Ingredients

1. **Rinse the Chickpeas**: Drain and thoroughly rinse the chickpeas to remove any excess liquid and prevent any strong "bean" taste.
2. **Soften the Dates**: If your dates are not soft, soak them in warm water for 10 minutes to make them easier to blend.

Blend the Base

1. **Blend Chickpeas and Dates**: In a food processor, combine the chickpeas, softened dates, and almond butter. Blend until the mixture becomes smooth and creamy. You may need to stop and scrape down the sides to ensure everything blends evenly.
2. **Add Oat Flour and Vanilla**: Add the oat flour and vanilla extract to the food processor. Blend again until it is well combined. The mixture should resemble a thick cookie dough. If the dough is too thick, add 1-2 tablespoons of almond milk to help with blending.

Fold in the Chocolate Chips

1. **Add Chocolate Chips**: Remove the dough from the food processor and transfer it to a bowl. Fold in the dark chocolate chips by hand, mixing them evenly throughout the dough.

Serve

- **Enjoy it Raw**: You can enjoy the chickpea cookie dough straight from the bowl! Use a spoon or roll the dough into bite-sized balls for easy snacking.
- **Optional Baking**: If you prefer baked cookies, preheat the oven to 350°F (175°C), scoop the dough into small rounds, and bake for 10-12 minutes until the edges are golden brown.

HEALING AND NUTRITION

This vegan chickpea cookie dough is not only a delicious snack but also a fantastic way to support a healthy lifestyle. The combination of chickpeas and oat flour provides fiber and plant-based protein, which helps to keep you feeling full and satisfied. Chickpeas are a low-glycemic food, meaning they will not spike blood sugar levels and help prevent energy crashes or excessive hunger.

One person who incorporated this recipe into their diet shared how it became a game-changer for them. They had been looking for healthier dessert options that did not rely on refined sugar or processed ingredients, and this chickpea cookie dough satisfied their sweet teeth while aligning with their weight loss goals. By replacing traditional cookie dough with this nutrient-dense alternative, they were able to curb their cravings for high-calorie sweets.

Over time, they noticed that the combination of fiber, healthy fats, and natural sweetness from the dates helped regulate their digestion, stabilize their energy levels, and support their weight loss efforts. In just three months, they lost 12 pounds while enjoying indulgent-tasting snacks like this one.

Dates, as a natural sweetener, are packed with vitamins, minerals, and antioxidants, and they provide energy without causing rapid blood sugar spikes. This recipe offers a delicious way to enjoy something sweet while staying on track with health goals, proving that you can indulge in desserts without compromising your well-being.

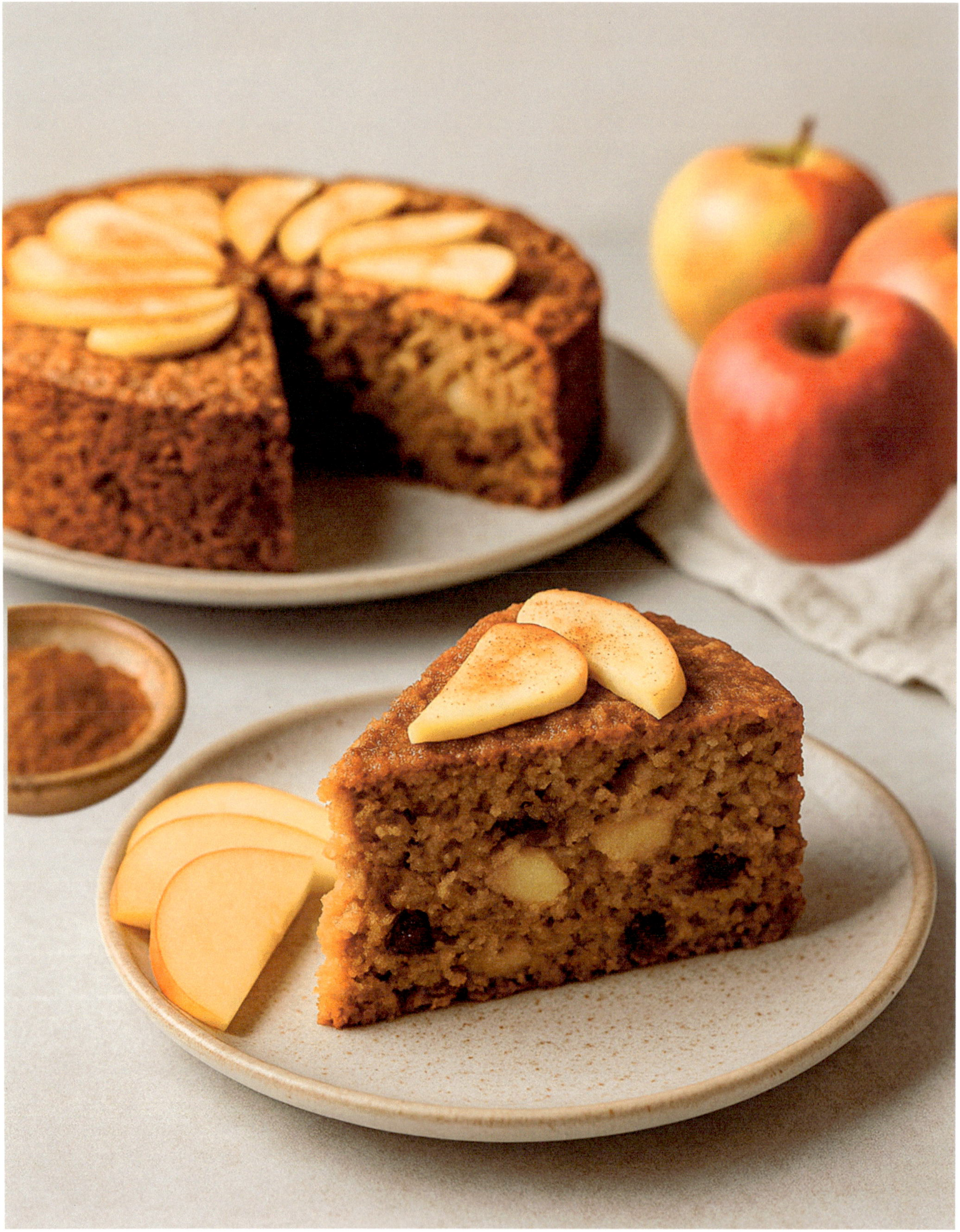

VEGAN APPLE CINNAMON CAKE RECIPE

This wholesome vegan apple cinnamon cake is naturally sweetened with bananas and raisins, full of fiber-rich oats, and spiced with cinnamon. Made without refined sugar or oil, this recipe is perfect for a healthy breakfast, snack, or dessert that satisfies cravings without compromising your health goals.

INGREDIENTS

- 2 medium apples (peeled and chopped)
- 2 cups of oats (blended into oat flour, or use store-bought oat flour)
- 1 ripe banana (mashed)
- 2 tbsp ground flaxseed (mixed with 5 tbsp water for a flax egg)
- Pinch of sea salt
- 2 tsp cinnamon
- 1 tbsp baking powder
- 1 tsp vanilla extract (optional)
- ¼ cup raisins
- ¼ cup almond milk or any plant-based milk (optional, for additional moisture)

INSTRUCTIONS

Prepare the Flax Egg

1. **Make the Flax Egg**: In a small bowl, mix 2 tablespoons of ground flaxseed with 5 tablespoons of water. Stir well and let it sit for 5-10 minutes to thicken. This will act as the egg replacement in the recipe.

Prepare the Apples and Oat Flour

1. **Chop the Apples**: Peel and chop the apples into small chunks, setting them aside for later.
2. **Make the Oat Flour**: If you are using rolled oats, blend them in a food processor or high-speed blender until they turn into a fine flour.

Mix the Dry Ingredients

1. **Combine Dry Ingredients**: In a large mixing bowl, combine the oat flour, cinnamon, baking powder, and a pinch of sea salt. Stir well to combine.

Mix the Wet Ingredients

1. **Mash the Banana**: In another bowl, mash the ripe banana until smooth.

2. **Add Flax Egg and Raisins**: Stir in the flax egg, raisins, and vanilla extract (if using) into the mashed banana mixture. Mix until well combined.
3. **Add the Wet to Dry**: Slowly add the wet mixture to the dry ingredients, stirring until a thick batter forms. If the batter seems too thick, you can add a little almond milk (or any plant-based milk) to reach a pourable consistency.

Fold in the Apples

1. **Add the Chopped Apples**: Gently fold the chopped apples into the batter until they are evenly distributed.

Bake the Cake

1. **Preheat the Oven**: Preheat your oven to 350°F (175°C).
2. **Prepare the Pan**: Lightly grease or line an 8-inch round cake pan (or loaf pan) with parchment paper.
3. **Pour and Bake**: Pour the batter into the prepared pan and smooth the top with a spatula. Bake for 30-35 minutes, or until a toothpick inserted into the center comes out clean and the top is golden brown.
4. **Cool**: Allow the cake to cool for 10-15 minutes in the pan before transferring it to a wire rack to cool completely.

Serve

Once cooled, slice and enjoy your vegan apple cinnamon cake. It pairs wonderfully with a cup of tea or coffee!

HEALING AND NUTRITION

This vegan apple cinnamon cake is not only a delicious, guilt-free treat but also a powerful tool in supporting a healthy lifestyle. The blend of fiber-rich oats, apples, and flaxseed makes this cake a great choice for those looking to manage their weight or improve digestion.

One person who regularly incorporated this recipe into their diet shared how it helped them achieve their weight loss goals. They had struggled with sugary, processed snacks that led to energy crashes and cravings, but this apple cinnamon cake provided a filling and nutritious alternative. The natural sweetness from bananas and raisins curbed their sweet tooth, while the oats and flaxseed kept them full longer.

Over the course of three months, they replaced high-calorie, refined sugar-filled desserts with this apple cinnamon cake and noticed significant changes in their energy levels and weight. By focusing on whole, plant-based ingredients like apples, oats, and flaxseed, they lost 15 pounds and saw improvements in their digestion. The high fiber content from oats and apples helped regulate their blood sugar levels, preventing spikes and crashes that often lead to overeating.

Incorporating this nutrient-dense cake into a balanced diet allowed them to indulge in something sweet while continuing on their healing journey. This recipe is a perfect example of how healthy ingredients can make a satisfying and delicious treat that contributes to overall well-being!

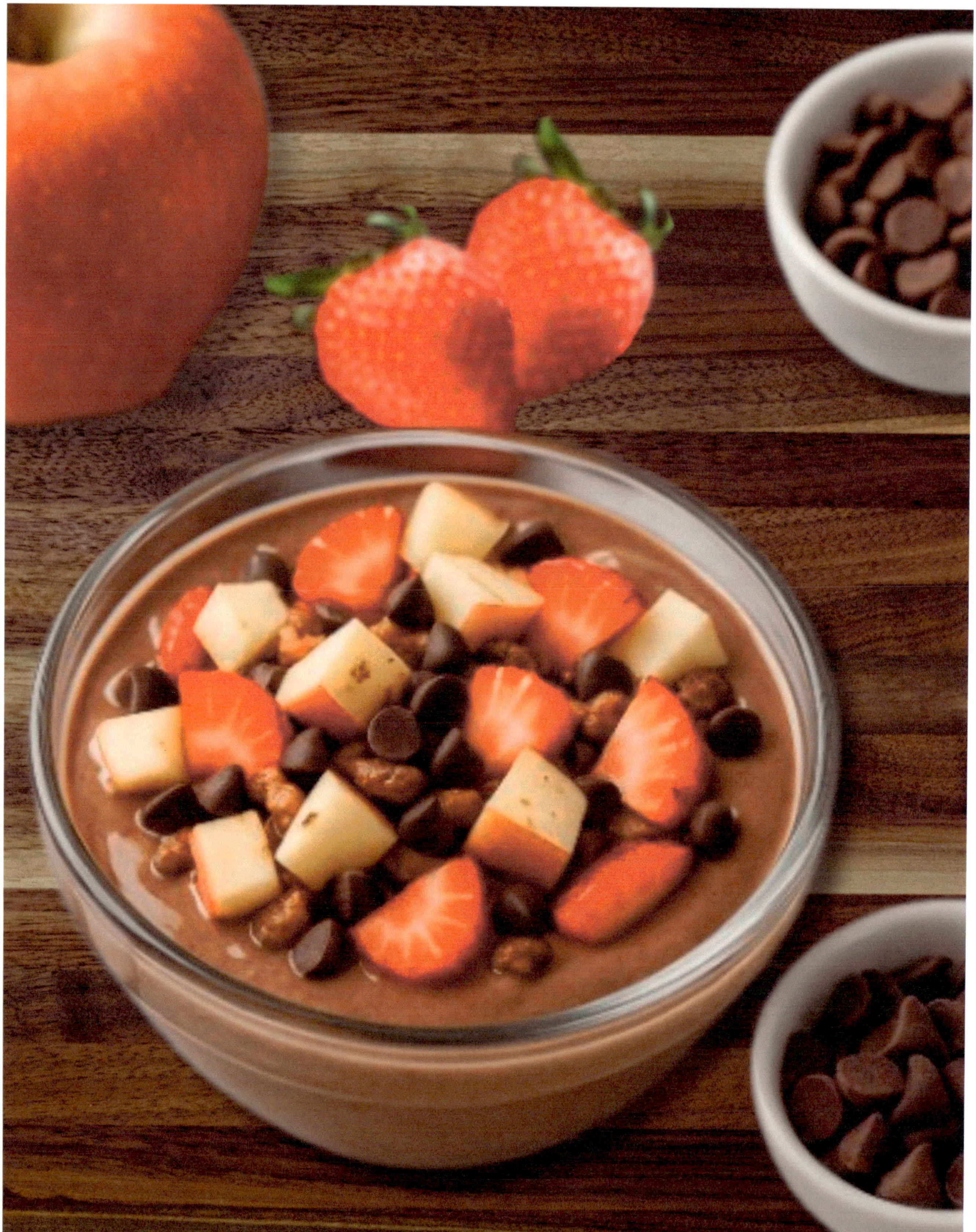

VEGAN APPLE CHOCOLATE YOGURT

This creamy, indulgent, yet healthy vegan yogurt recipe combines the rich flavor of chocolate, the sweetness of strawberries, and the freshness of apples. It is a perfect balance of wholesome ingredients, ideal for a snack, dessert, or even breakfast. Packed with antioxidants and healthy fats, it also supports healing and weight loss.

INGREDIENTS:

- 1 cup of vegan yogurt (coconut, almond, or soy-based)
- 1/4 cup vegan chocolate chips (dark or semi-sweet)
- 1 small apple (diced)
- 4-5 fresh strawberries (sliced)
- 1 tablespoon coconut oil
- 1 tablespoon maple syrup or agave (optional for sweetness)
- 1/2 teaspoon cinnamon (optional for added flavor)

INSTRUCTIONS:

Prepare the Chocolate Sauce:

- In a small saucepan, melt the coconut oil over low heat.
- Add the vegan chocolate chips to the melted coconut oil and stir continuously until the chocolate is fully melted and smooth. Set aside to cool slightly.

Prepare the Apples:

- Wash and dice the apple into small bite-sized pieces. You can leave the skin on for added fiber and nutrients.

Layer the Vegan Yogurt:

- In a medium-sized bowl or serving dish, add 1 cup of vegan yogurt as the base. You can use any plant-based yogurt, but coconut or almond yogurt pairs well with this recipe.

Add Apple and Strawberries:

- Evenly spread the diced apple pieces over the top of the yogurt.
- Add the sliced strawberries to the dish, arranging them on top or mixing them with the apple.

Drizzle the Chocolate Sauce:

- Once the melted chocolate has cooled slightly, drizzle it over the yogurt, apples, and strawberries. You can also swirl the chocolate through the yogurt for a marbled effect.

Sweeten (Optional):

- If you want a sweeter taste, drizzle 1 tablespoon of maple syrup or agave syrup over the top.
- Optionally, sprinkle a pinch of cinnamon for an extra flavor boost.

Serve:

- Enjoy immediately as a fresh, decadent snack, or chill in the refrigerator for 10-15 minutes if you prefer it cold.

HEALING AND NUTRITION

This vegan apple chocolate yogurt recipe has helped me achieve both wellness and weight management goals while still enjoying something delicious. Here is a testimony from someone who has experienced its benefits:

TESTIMONIAL: "*I was looking for a healthy snack that felt indulgent, and this recipe became my go-to. The combination of fresh fruits, yogurt, and chocolate made me feel satisfied, and it curbed my sweet cravings without derailing my weight loss efforts. The coconut oil helped boost my metabolism, while the fiber from the apples and the antioxidants from the chocolate contributed to better digestion and skin health. By eating this regularly as an afternoon snack, I felt more energized, and it became easier to manage my weight. It is truly a guilt-free treat that keeps me full and healthy.*"

Health Benefits:

- **Vegan Yogurt**: A probiotic-rich ingredient that supports gut health and aids digestion, which can contribute to weight loss.
- **Coconut Oil**: Contains medium-chain triglycerides (MCTs) that are known to boost metabolism, provide energy, and support fat burning.
- **Apples**: High in fiber, which keeps you full longer and supports digestion, making it easier to manage your appetite.
- **Vegan Chocolate Chips**: Dark chocolate is rich in antioxidants, and when used in moderation, it can promote heart health and reduce cravings.

This delicious vegan yogurt dish can help you stay on track with your wellness goals, all while feeling like a special treat.

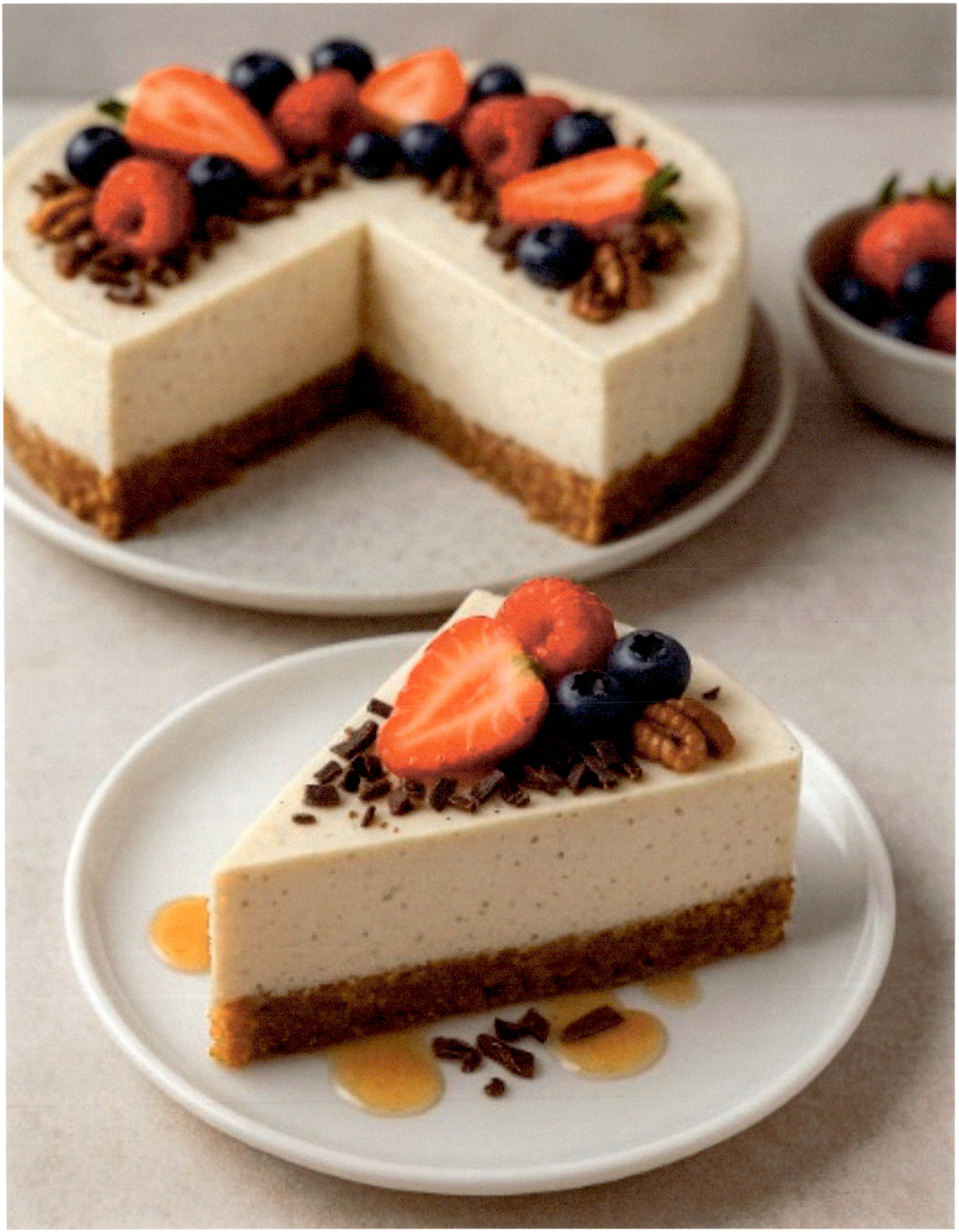

CHEESECAKE WITH FLAXSEED

AND VEGAN CREAM CHEESE

INGREDIENTS:

- 1 1/2 cups graham cracker crumbs (or gluten-free alternative)
- 1/4 cup of coconut oil (melted)
- 1/4 cup of water (for flaxseed mixture)
- 2 cups of vegan cream cheese
- 1 tablespoon ground flaxseed (for binding)
- 1/2 cup maple syrup or agave syrup (for sweetness)
- 1 cup organic vegan cream cheese
- 1 tablespoon lemon juice (for tartness)
- 1 teaspoon vanilla extract

INSTRUCTIONS:

Prepare the Flaxseed Mixture (Flax "Egg")

1. In a small bowl, combine 1 tablespoon of ground flaxseed with 1/4 cup of water.
2. Stir well and let it sit for about 10-15 minutes until it forms a gel-like consistency. This acts as a binding agent and replaces the need for eggs in the cheesecake filling.

Prepare the Crust

1. In a mixing bowl, combine the graham cracker crumbs with the melted coconut oil.
2. Stir until the mixture resembles wet sand.
3. Press the mixture into the bottom of an 8-inch or 9-inch springform pan to form the crust.
4. Place the pan in the refrigerator to set while preparing the filling.

Make the Vegan Cheesecake Filling

1. In a large bowl, combine the vegan cream cheese and organic vegan cream cheese.
2. Using a hand mixer (or stand mixer), beat the cream cheese until smooth and creamy.
3. Add the maple syrup or agave syrup, lemon juice, and vanilla extract. Mix until well combined.
4. Stir in the flaxseed mixture (flax "egg") to bind the filling.
5. Beat the mixture for another 1-2 minutes until everything is smooth and creamy.

Assemble the Cheesecake

1. Remove the crust from the refrigerator and pour the cheesecake filling evenly over the prepared crust.
2. Smooth the top with a spatula to create an even surface.

Chill the Cheesecake

1. Place the cheesecake in the refrigerator and let it chill for at least 4-6 hours, or overnight, to set completely. This allows the flavors to meld and the texture to firm up.

Serve and Enjoy

1. Once the cheesecake is fully chilled and set, carefully remove the springform pan.
2. Slice and serve your creamy, delicious vegan cheesecake.

Optional Toppings:

- Fresh berries (strawberries, raspberries, blueberries)
- Shaved vegan chocolate
- A drizzle of maple syrup or agave

HEALING AND NUTRITION

This vegan cheesecake has been a game-changer for those looking to indulge in a sweet treat without compromising their health goals. Flaxseed, one of the key ingredients, is rich in fiber, omega-3 fatty acids, and antioxidants, which promote heart health and aid digestion. Many people who have integrated flaxseed into their diets find it helps curb cravings and contributes to a feeling of fullness, supporting weight management.

The absence of dairy in this cheesecake makes it a lighter alternative to traditional cheesecake, significantly reducing unhealthy fats. By using vegan cream cheese and organic ingredients, individuals have reported experiencing less bloating and inflammation compared to consuming conventional dairy products.

This vegan cheesecake has also been popular among those on healing diets, as it allows for a guilt-free dessert while maintaining nutritional benefits. It has helped many on their weight-loss journeys by offering a low-sugar, nutrient-dense alternative to conventional desserts.

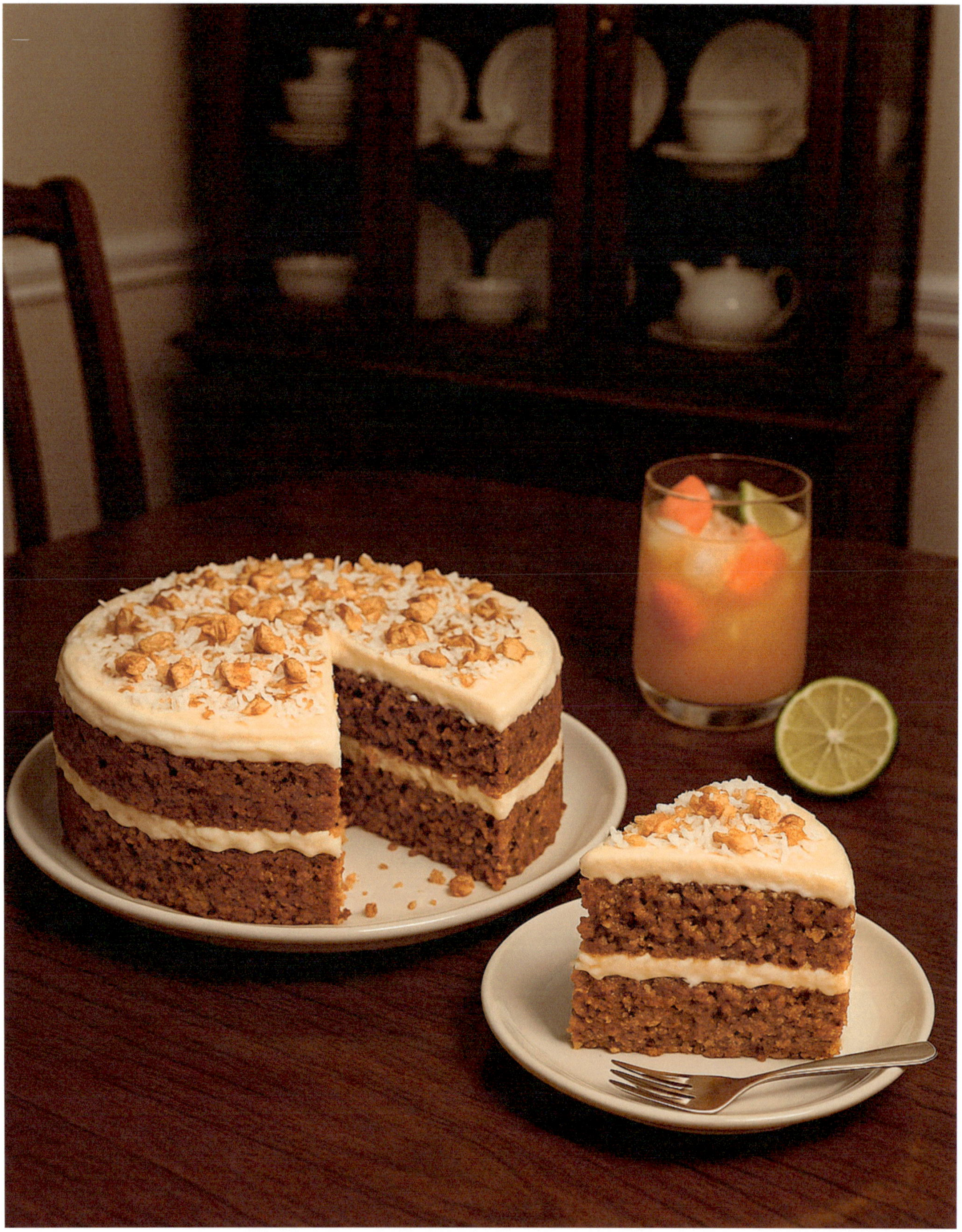

VEGAN CARROT CAKE

with Coconut, Oats and Dates

INGREDIENTS:

For the Cake:

- 1 1/2 cups grated carrots
- 1 cup rolled oats (ground into flour)
- 1/2 cup shredded coconut (unsweetened)
- 1 cup pitted dates (soaked for 10 minutes in warm water)
- 1/2 cup walnut flakes (or chopped walnuts)
- 1 teaspoon ground cinnamon
- 1/2 teaspoon ground ginger
- 1 teaspoon vanilla extract
- 1/2 cup cashew milk (or any other plant-based milk)

For the Frosting (optional):

- 1 cup-soaked cashews (soaked for 4 hours or overnight)
- 2 tablespoons maple syrup or agave
- 1/4 cup of coconut milk
- 1 teaspoon vanilla extract
- 1 tablespoon lemon juice

INSTRUCTIONS:

Prepare the Ingredients

1. Preheat the oven to 350°F (175°C) and line a cake pan (8-inch round or square) with parchment paper or lightly grease it with coconut oil.
2. Soak the pitted dates in warm water for 10 minutes to soften them for easier blending.
3. Grate the carrots and set them aside.

Make the Oat Flour

1. Place 1 cup of rolled oats in a blender or food processor and blend until they turn into a fine flour-like consistency.
2. Set the oat flour aside for later.

Make the Date Paste

1. Drain the soaked dates and place them in a food processor or blender.
2. Blend until they form a smooth paste. If necessary, add a little water (from the soaking) to reach a smooth texture.

Mix the Dry Ingredients

1. In a large bowl, combine the oat flour, shredded coconut, walnut flakes, cinnamon, and ginger.
2. Stir well to ensure all dry ingredients are evenly distributed.

Combine Wet Ingredients

1. In a separate bowl, mix the grated carrots, date paste, cashew milk, and vanilla extract.
2. Stir until the wet ingredients are well combined.

Create the Batter

1. Pour the wet mixture into the bowl with the dry ingredients.
2. Stir everything together until it is fully combined. The batter should be thick and sticky.
3. If it feels too dry, add a little more cashew milk, 1 tablespoon at a time.

Bake the Cake

1. Pour the batter into the prepared cake pan and spread it evenly.
2. Bake in the preheated oven for 30-35 minutes, or until a toothpick inserted into the center comes out clean.
3. Once baked, remove the cake from the oven and let it cool in the pan for 10-15 minutes. Then transfer to a cooling rack to cool completely.

Prepare the Cashew Frosting (Optional)

1. Drain the soaked cashews and blend them in a food processor with the maple syrup, coconut milk, vanilla extract, and lemon juice.
2. Blend until smooth and creamy. If necessary, add a little more coconut milk to achieve the desired consistency.
3. Once the cake is fully cooled, spread the frosting evenly over the top.

Serve and Enjoy

1. Slice and serve your moist and delicious vegan carrot cake.
2. Optionally, sprinkle some extra walnut flakes or shredded coconut on top for added texture and presentation.

HEALING AND NUTRITION

This vegan carrot cake has been celebrated not just for its flavor but for its nourishing properties as well. The use of whole-food ingredients such as **dates**, **walnuts**, and **oats** makes this cake naturally sweetened and high in fiber, which supports digestion and helps regulate blood sugar levels, making it a guilt-free dessert option for those on a weight-loss journey.

Carrots, rich in vitamins A and C, provide antioxidant benefits, aiding in healing and boosting immunity. The **fiber** from oats, walnuts, and dates helps keep you feeling full longer, curbing unnecessary snacking and promoting healthy digestion which are key factors in managing weight effectively.

Many people have shared how switching to desserts like this vegan carrot cake has allowed them to enjoy sweet treats without compromising their health goals. The absence of refined sugars and flour, combined with nutrient-dense ingredients, has supported individuals not only in losing weight but also in feeling more energetic and balanced.

Additionally, this recipe avoids dairy and animal-based products, reducing inflammation and promoting a heart-healthy lifestyle, making it ideal for those aiming for long-term well-being and sustainable weight management.

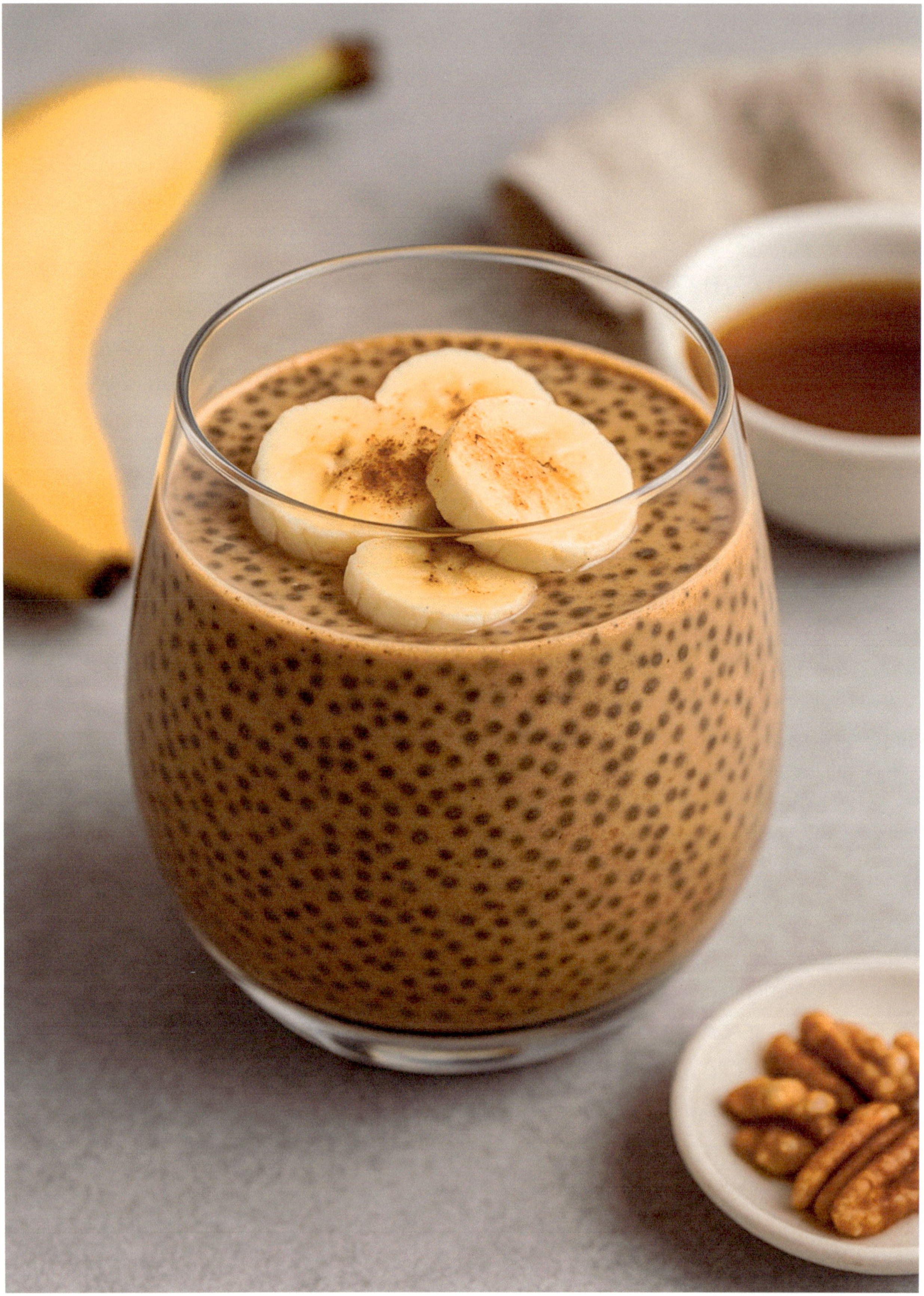

VEGAN CHIA BANANA COFFEE PUDDING

INGREDIENTS:

- 1/4 cup chia seeds
- 1 ripe banana
- 1/2 cup brewed coffee (cooled)
- 1/2 cup coconut milk
- 1/2 cup almond milk
- 2 tablespoons maple syrup (or to taste)
- 1 teaspoon vanilla extract
- 1/4 cup water (optional, for thinning the pudding)

INSTRUCTIONS:

Prepare the Chia Base

1. In a mixing bowl, combine the chia seeds, coconut milk, almond milk, coffee, and maple syrup.
2. Stir well to ensure the chia seeds are evenly distributed throughout the liquid mixture.
3. Let the mixture sit for about 5-10 minutes, then stir again to prevent the chia seeds from clumping together.

Blend the Banana

1. In a separate bowl, mash the ripe banana until smooth.
2. Add the vanilla extract to the mashed banana and mix well.

Combine Banana and Chia Mixture

1. After the chia mixture has thickened slightly, stir in the mashed banana mixture.
2. Mix well until the banana is evenly incorporated into the chia mixture.
3. If the pudding seems too thick, add a little water to reach your desired consistency, but remember that chia seeds will continue to absorb liquid as they sit.

Let It Set

1. Cover the bowl with plastic wrap or transfer the mixture to individual jars or bowls.
2. Place it in the refrigerator to set for at least 3-4 hours or overnight for best results. The chia seeds will swell and create a thick, pudding-like texture.

Serve and Enjoy

1. Once the chia pudding has set, give it a good stir before serving.
2. Optionally, you can top it with additional banana slices, a sprinkle of cinnamon, or a drizzle of maple syrup for extra sweetness.

HEALING AND NUTRITION

This chia banana coffee pudding offers a blend of energizing ingredients that support both healing and weight management. **Chia seeds** are packed with fiber, omega-3 fatty acids, and antioxidants, making them a superfood that helps regulate digestion, balance blood sugar levels, and promote satiety. This helps with curbing cravings, making it easier for people to manage their weight.

Bananas provide natural sweetness, potassium, and essential vitamins, while also promoting good digestion and heart health. Combined with **coffee**, which adds a gentle energy boost and enhances metabolism, this pudding is a satisfying yet light option for breakfast or a snack.

Many people find that incorporating chia seeds into their diet improves digestive health and supports sustained weight loss, as it keeps them feeling fuller longer. The use of plant-based milks like **coconut milk** and **almond milk** keeps this recipe dairy-free, reducing inflammation and supporting a more balanced lifestyle.

This pudding not only satisfies sweet cravings but also nourishes the body, making it an ideal treat for those seeking a dessert with health benefits. By cutting out refined sugars and opting for **maple syrup** as a natural sweetener, this pudding is lower in glycemic impact, further supporting weight loss and overall well-being.

CONCLUSION

Choosing a plant-based lifestyle is one of the most powerful commitments a person can make to their health and well-being. It is not just about what is on the plate. It is about redefining the relationship with food, making conscious choices, and embracing a way of eating that supports both the body and mind. The foods we choose today shape how we feel tomorrow, influencing everything from energy levels to mental clarity and long-term vitality. This journey is about more than personal health; it is about building a lifestyle that fosters longevity, sustainability, and a greater connection to the natural world. Every meal is an opportunity to nourish, to strengthen, and to create lasting habits that will benefit not only ourselves but those around us. There is power in knowing that what we consume has a direct impact on how we show up in the world, physically, emotionally, and even spiritually.

Transitioning to a plant-based lifestyle may seem overwhelming at first, but every small step makes a difference. It is not about perfection; it is about consistency and a willingness to learn. Exploring new foods, experimenting with different flavors, and understanding how to create balanced meals can turn eating into a joyful, fulfilling experience rather than a routine or obligation. By approaching this lifestyle with curiosity rather than restriction, it becomes a journey of discovery rather than sacrifice. This is also about creating a lasting impact. When we make intentional choices about food, we inspire those around us to do the same. Families, friends, and communities benefit when we share knowledge, recipes, and the joy of eating well. A plant-based lifestyle is not just about personal gain; it is about reshaping generational habits, improving overall wellness, and cultivating a mindset that values nourishment as an essential part of life.

For those considering this path, know that it does not have to be an all-or-nothing shift. Small changes, like adding more whole foods, reducing processed ingredients, and incorporating more plant-based meals, can have a profound effect. The key is to move at a comfortable pace, staying open to learning and evolving along the way. The goal is not just to change how we eat but to enhance how we live. Ultimately, food is one of the most powerful tools we have for improving our health, our mindset, and our future. Embracing a plant-based lifestyle is not just a dietary choice; it is a commitment to self-care, sustainability, and intentional living. It is about experiencing food as a source of healing, joy, and nourishment in its purest form. By making thoughtful, informed decisions about what we put on our plates, we empower ourselves to live more vibrant, fulfilling lives. This is not just about eating differently, it is about living better.

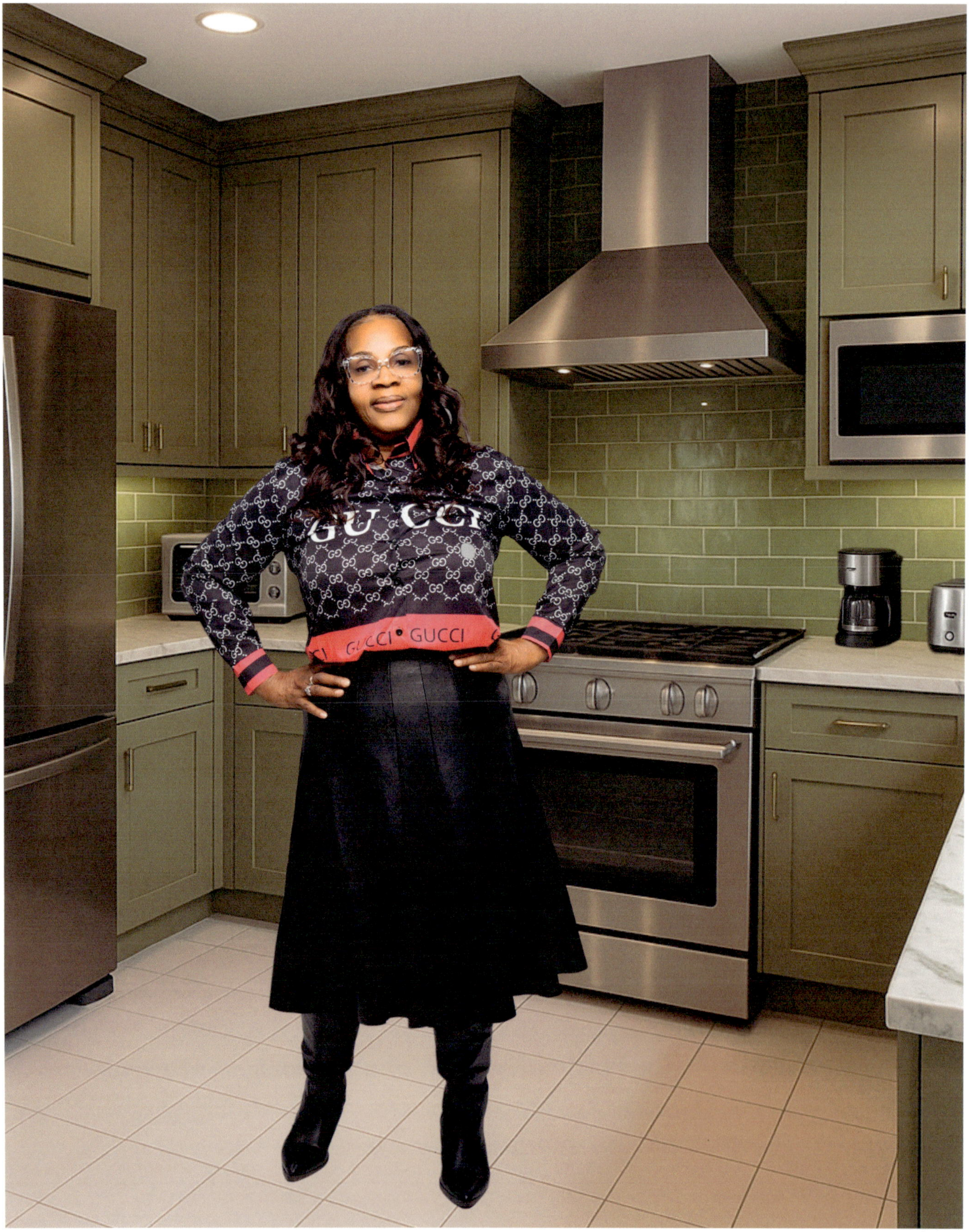
GUCCI
GUCCI • GUCCI

Closing Message from the Author

As we come to the end of 'From The Ground,' I hope these recipes inspire you to continue your journey toward health and wholeness, rooted in the abundance of the earth. Every meal is an opportunity to nourish both body and spirit, and may your choices reflect the beauty of creation that God has given us. Just as the scriptures remind us, "I have given you every herb bearing seed, which is upon the face of all the earth" (Genesis 1:29, KJV), let these plant-based dishes bring you life and vitality. Remember, healing begins from within, and what you feed your body is an act of love and care. May you be blessed with wellness, joy, and strength in every bite.

Thank you for letting nature's bounty feed your soul and heal your body from the inside out.

— Mechille Renee Tate-Akinkuotu

Made in the USA
Monee, IL
05 November 2026

67383132R00093